POLIO :

THE ERADICATION IMBROGLIO

The Malady & its Remedy

T Jacob John & Dhanya Dharmapalan

NOTION PRESS

NOTION PRESS

India. Singapore. Malaysia.

Published by Notion Press 2021

ISBN 9781638063650

Disclaimer

The views expressed in this book are solely the personal views and findings of the authors. The people, institutions or organisations that authors may be affiliated with in any manner, have not endorsed such views / findings and no such endorsement shall be construed unless specified otherwise in the book.

Although the authors have made every effort to ensure that the information in this book was correct at time of publication, the authors do not assume and hereby disclaim any liability to any party for any loss, damage, or disruption caused by errors or omissions, whether such errors or omissions result from negligence, accident, or any other cause.

Credit

Cover Design Copyright © 2021 by T Jacob John and Dhanya Dharmapalan

Cover page images

Left: An ancient Egyptian carving of a man with right leg showing muscle-wasting, shortening and equinus deformity of foot. He needed a stick as support for walking. (Source: Wikipedia, CC BY SA-3.0; https://creativecommons.org/licenses/by-sa/3.0/)

Right: A young boy in India showing the very same features on his left side. The photo, taken from behind, reminds us that we can make polio walk away from us, into the sunset. (Photo, Courtesy: Vipin Vashishtha).

CONTENTS

Preface

Vaccines are powerful tools in human mastery over microbes causing diseases. They are used in medical practice to prevent diseases in individuals, as vaccines induce protective immunity in vaccinated individuals. This is vaccination as preventive medicine.

By vaccinating a large proportion of individuals, the transmission dynamics of microbes that are human-to-human transmitted, gets altered. The result is a declining disease burden not only in the vaccinated segment of the population but also in the unvaccinated segment. Community-wide vaccination is a tool in public health for disease control. The visible effect of disease reduction is actually the result of the invisible effect of slowing down the transmission of the microbe. The extreme form of control is stopping transmission altogether in the community. When the transmission is interrupted in an entire country, we say that the infection is eliminated. Infection may get imported from outside any time. However, if all countries eliminate infection, there is no source for importation, and that is the principle of global eradication of infection.

A global agenda to eradicate must be binding on all countries. The United Nations (UN) bring all countries to the table. Health matters are dealt with the World Health Organisation (WHO), which is a UN Agency. The forum in which all Ministers of Health are enrolled is the World Health Assembly (WHA) with its secretariat at WHO. In 1966 the WHA resolved by majority vote to eradicate smallpox for which a highly efficacious smallpox vaccine was available. The time target was 10 years, and it was accomplished in 11 years. The next disease eradication resolution was unanimously passed in 1988 – to eradicate polio, and its time target was a bit more liberal, 12 years.

The confidence of WHA for success in 12 years was due to the facts that in countries that still had polio, it occurred almost exclusively in under-five children and that a vaccination platform had already been established in all such countries -- the Expanded Program on Immunization(EPI) to target specifically under-five children. Smallpox was not age-restricted but could occur at any age. Its eradication was a formidable task since no vaccination platform was available. The EPI was launched only as the smallpox eradication was nearing completion. The world was truly ready for polio eradication.

For polio, two vaccines were available -- the inactivated poliovirus vaccine, IPV, and live attenuated oral poliovirus vaccine, OPV. All about the two vaccines, their pluses and minuses, were well studied and documented by the time EPI was established. In 1988 additional information about the vaccines was available from 14 years of EPI experience -- its successes and failures.

We are now in 2020, twenty years past the eradication target year of 2000. The new millennium of twenty-first century was promised to be totally polio-free. Success has eluded the polio eradication program for twenty years. The target year was revised first as 2005, and later to new target years, and having failed repeatedly, we are in 2020 with no light at the end of the tunnel. The reason for this fiasco is a simple error – the tactical choice of only one of the two vaccines, namely OPV, and stubborn insistence on its exclusive use.

The two vaccines IPV and OPV have contrasting characteristics that were well-known by 1988. The eradication program, instead of following the WHA Resolution in letter and spirit, to use both vaccines, unilaterally decided to use OPV exclusively for eradication. That choice had no backing of science or biomedical ethics, but only the belief of the program leaders that OPV alone should be used to eradicate polio. The justification for the exclusive use of OPV was perhaps the fact that in 1974 the EPI had recommended to all countries to use OPV exclusively. By 1988, with fourteen years of experience, EPI could not control polio using OPV in low and middle income countries and that was the main reason for the WHA resolution for the global eradication of polio.

In 1988 polio experts knew clearly that IPV was completely safe and exquisitely efficacious. They also knew that OPV was neither highly efficacious in the low-middle income countries that were struggling to control polio, nor completely safe in any country. Too many children were developing polio in spite of taking the recommended three or five or even seven doses of OPV. Insisting on eradication using it exclusively appeared to be an attempt to prove that OPV was the right choice. But why, who was interested in protecting the reputation of OPV? By 1988 experts knew that there were also major safety problems with OPV.

That its use, let alone exclusive use, was contravening public health ethics, as it was by itself a cause of polio paralysis, did not move the program leadership to put eradication as the only goal, not protecting the reputation of OPV and justifying the choice of OPV by EPI. As an embarrassing consequence, in 2019, two countries still had polio due to natural wild virus, but nineteen had program-caused polio due to OPV. In 2019, the number of OPV-caused polio outnumbered wild virus polio by about 150 per cent. In 2020, the number of countries with wild virus polio remains two, but 25 countries had OPV-caused polio, the cases outnumbering natural cases by over 600 per cent.

We write this book to declare: enough is enough. Let us get on with polio eradication – both wild virus polio and OPV-caused polio, by using the other vaccine, IPV, and learn how to use it under best tactics for success. We present our reasoning for the promise of success by applying principles of public health, vaccine science, disease epidemiology and biomedical ethics.

The munificent donor countries and organizations must insist on accountability of the program. Since the year 2000, annually about one billion US dollars are spent on the eradication program. Global public health leaders must insist on equity in sharing both benefits and risks of interventions. We have created an inequitable world with some countries having full freedom from natural polio and OPV-induced polio while others are burdened with hundreds of children getting paralyzed by the misguided program policy.

We owe this obligation to lend our voices to the voiceless children getting polio paralysis for no fault of theirs or their parents. We appeal to public leaders of the world to lend their voices in solidarity with them. The roadmap to the finishing line is clearly drawn and presented in this book. We hope the program leaders will relent and take the path of science and ethics with wisdom.

§§§

Parable

In 1986, Rotary International sent me as an envoy to Somalia to prepare the health ministry to receive and utilize a PolioPlus grant for polio vaccination of all under-five children for five years. The return flight got delayed, and I sat in the waiting lounge of the Mogadishu airport. The tarmac was in view through a large glass pane. Suddenly I noticed a spider jump at a fly that had just landed near the spider. You know jumping spiders do not spin a web to catch prey but jump on insects in a split second.

The spider missed the catch; the fly flew away. I thought in my mind: smart fly. Then another fly landed near the spider – the spider jumped, but it missed again. I thought: dumb spider. I sat watching the spider jump at a third fly and missing once again.

I recalled the old story of the spider and Robert Bruce. The Scottish king was defeated in battle, and he escaped and hid in a cave, dejected and dispirited. He observed a spider jumping from one side at the mouth of the cave to reach the other side, hanging with its thread that prevented it from falling to the ground – but it failed. It scrambled back up and jumped again, and missed again. The king watched the spider jump and fail again and again. It did not give up. On the seventh attempt the spider succeeded. He learned the lesson: try and try again until you succeed. Robert Bruce regrouped his men and won the next battle. So mentally I gave my spider seven attempts to succeed.

But that need not be the right way in other situations. The spider knew that success was possible from experience and was right. The jumping spider failed the seventh, eighth, ninth and tenth attempts. With curiosity I got up, walked closer and took a look at the spider – lo and behold, the spider was inside but all the flies were outside. There was a glass wall between them. Try and try again lesson applied only if the flies were on the same side with the spider.

Is this not true in life on many occasions? Everything is not as it seems to be. We often miss the glass wall between where action is needed and where action is applied. When we fail we find all sorts of excuses but fail to perceive the invisible glass as the real reason. There is an old saying that man is the only animal that fails to learn from experience. Did not Einstein say that doing the same thing over and over again, expecting a different result is insanity? So, people do repeat action that failed repeatedly but fail to learn the reason and to modify the action.

Have you ever wondered why? Ben Vermaercke in Leuven found that rats performed better than humans in some experiments that required decision based on pattern showed earlier. He explained the reason: there are two ways to apply the lesson from one situation to another. That choice may be rule-based or by 'information integration'. Rule-based learning is an evolutionary development in humans. Vermaercke postulated that humans, faced with specific data points, tend to apply a learned rule and get it all wrong. In simple tasks, rats were better at information integration as they had no rules to apply. Humans tend to become enslaved by rules, dogmas, and beliefs and fail to integrate complex information to arrive at the right solutions.

T Jacob John

§§§

Section One

The World Health Organisation is a special agency of the United Nations, to address public health issues globally. Its headquarters is in Geneva, Switzerland. Among its many defined objectives are the following: to act as the directing and coordinating authority on international health work, and to stimulate and advance work to eradicate epidemic, endemic and other diseases.

Outstanding achievements of WHO include, among many others, the establishment and promotion of the Expanded Program on Immunization in 1974 and the eradication of smallpox in 1977 and its certification in 1979.

As a natural outcome of increasing ambition, enhanced capacity and emerging opportunities, the goal of polio eradication was set in 1988, to gift a polio-free world to the children of the twenty-first century. Eradication was to be achieved in 2000, so that no child born thereafter should develop polio. As we write in 2020, the goal set for 2000 has not yet been reached. Even its finishing line is not yet in sight.

The following three chapters will set the stage for the drama of the dream turning nightmare.

1. DECLARING WAR ON POLIO: REVISITING THE RESOLUTION

Go to war only if you are sure to win. Plan strategy, tactics and logistics in the War Room. Do not declare war without full preparation.

Every sign was positive for resolving, in 1988, to eradicate polio. Measles was also a worthy target. For every child paralyzed by polio, one child was killed by measles. The then epidemiology of both infections was quite similar, essentially affecting children below five years. Both diseases should and could have been targeted for eradication since immunizing children with vaccines was the common strategy for both. Clinical and virological surveillance was needed for both. Very high immunization coverage was necessary for both. Every child had to be contacted and vaccinated – against one disease or two diseases? Why not two?

If measles eradication was targeted, the measles vaccine would have been the intervention tool. The measles vaccine is given in many countries as a combined measles-mumps-rubella (MMR) vaccine. Measles and rubella surveillance could be easily combined as fever and rash surveillance. So measles and rubella could be eradicated together. Mumps would probably not be eradicated, as immunity induced by mumps vaccine is not as robust and long-lasting as that of measles and rubella. But mumps could be controlled.

Some countries use a combined measles-rubella (MR) vaccine. Eradication of polio, measles and rubella required vaccine coverage of 95% or more of infants and very young children. Vaccines against polio, measles and rubella can be given to all the children reached. Two or three doses of IPV and two or three doses of MR (or MMR) vaccine would have been enough and could have been given to all children reached for eradicating either polio and measles or measles and rubella. That would have been a desirable proposition. But that was not to be; vision, imagination, compassion and courage of conviction were lacking.

When everyone has to do the job already assigned, who was there to develop a new idea and work out all details? New ideas ought to come from the highest leadership. Visionary leaders are those who watch the world and read the signs of the times. But that is not how it happened. Several 'external' events had pushed the agenda for polio eradication. Pushed is the right word, since the system was not quite ready for it.

Great lessons from smallpox eradication

WHO was actually well experienced in the concept and management of eradication, with the war trophy of smallpox eradication already in its bag, a decade earlier. The war on smallpox began with a World Health Assembly (WHA) Resolution for global smallpox eradication, passed by majority (not unanimous) vote, in 1966. In October 1977, the world's last case of endemic smallpox was documented – less than 11 years from the start. The program target of 10 years was missed only by nine months and 26 days. In May 1980, the WHA declared "*the world and all its peoples have won freedom from* smallpox."[1]

The strategy was straightforward: smallpox vaccination, until all smallpox was prevented. The tactics included surveillance to detect every reported or rumored case of smallpox and interrupting further spread by vaccinating all susceptible persons around. Look-alike diseases had to be excluded by laboratory tests. Tactics and logistics were tailored to fit each country. There was a commander-in-chief for the war.

Expanded Program on Immunization and beyond

The phenomenal progress of smallpox eradication by the early 1970s illustrated the power of immunization in the global public health agenda, not merely for disease prevention in individuals. There was a need to promote more extensive use of several under-utilized vaccines in developing countries that were without organized public health departments and universal primary healthcare. WHO designed and launched the Expanded Program on Immunization (EPI) in 1974. In concept, EPI was the bridge between 'horizontal' universal primary healthcare and 'vertical' tool-based intervention targeting a few diseases, otherwise known as 'selective disease control'. Ideally, the two could have been established together each reinforcing the other. In reality, the two became competing concepts for public health leaders.

DA Henderson who directed the smallpox eradication program in its final phase had stated: "*Soon after the [1980] Assembly, I was angrily confronted by a senior WHO official who spoke slowly and deliberately, 'Let me assure you that in this organisation, there will never again be a vertical programme such as smallpox eradication.' A prevalent view was that categorical programmes like smallpox or malaria eradication were major impediments to the development of basic healthcare systems, luring governments into extravagant, futile campaigns that compromised existing health programmes."* [1]

The decade of the 1980s was available for setting new goals of climbing higher mountain peaks – but that was also a period of vacillation.

In 1978 the Alma Ata Declaration created the agenda for WHO to take primary healthcare forward and make it universal. The declaration emerged out of an International Conference on Primary Healthcare, held in Alma Ata in USSR (now Almaty in Khazakstan), 6-12 September, 1978.

A competing concept and agenda came from two experts in the Rockefeller Institute in New York, in 1979, in a publication in the New England Journal of Medicine, under the title: Selective Primary Health Care: an interim strategy for disease control in developing countries.[2] The global health management atmosphere was vitiated by the philosophy of 'selective primary healthcare' – a euphemism for vertical control of a few selected diseases, essentially tuberculosis and malaria. Its promotional argument was its emphasis on the cost-effectiveness of vertical programs with measurable results. KW Newell stated succinctly and sharply: "The advocates of highly selected and specific health interventions have ignored, or put on one side, the ideas which are at the core of what could be described as the primary health care revolution."[3]

EPI, launched in 1974, had targeted '6 killer diseases' for prevention and control. The decade of 1980s was ideal for a grand vision of combining all lessons from smallpox eradication and EPI, and target measles and polio, the two virus diseases among the six EPI targets, for simultaneous eradication. They met all biological criteria for eradication – the extreme version of control.

That was not to be. Unfortunately, even the actual execution of EPI became vertical, without helping developing countries understand the importance of formal public health departments and universal primary healthcare.[4] Instead of being a means to disease control, EPI was seen by the top leadership (both in WHO and in developing countries) as an end in itself.

In most countries of three WHO Regions, EPI was performing well – they had understood the importance of public health and universal healthcare. They were the Regions of the Americas, Europe and the Western Pacific. There were reasons for it. The remaining three Regions – South East Asia, Africa and the Eastern Mediterranean had many countries not doing well with EPI. There must have been reasons for it. Did anyone explore?

The message was clear: one size would not fit all. The very last countries to stop smallpox were in the Regions of SE Asia and Africa. The battle terrains were not level. Tactics had to be tailor-made.

Forces that pushed WHO into the drafting of Resolution

The Rotary International had launched its PolioPlus program in 1985, to immunize all under-five children of the world against polio for full five years by Rotary's centenary year of 2005. Pan American Health Organisation (PAHO), the Regional Branch of WHO, had resolved in 1986, assured of fund support from PolioPlus, to eliminate polio by 1990 in the Region of Americas.

Thereafter the WHO Regional Offices of Europe and Western Pacific had resolved to emulate PAHO and eliminate polio by the year 2000. The WHA Resolution had noted this – "...that poliomyelitis is the target disease most amenable to global eradication, and that regional eradication goals by or before the year 2000 have already been set in the Regions of the Americas, Europe and the Western Pacific." When three Regions wanted polio eliminated, and were moving forward, with targets of 1990 (PAHO) and 2000 (Regions of Europe and Western Pacific), what should the WHO headquarters do? How would WHO look, in the eyes of the world? How could WHO look at public health leaders in their eyes?

The Task Force for Child Survival, established by US Past President Jimmy Carter, had convened a meeting in Talloires, France, 10-12 March 1988: "Protecting the World's Children – an agenda for the 1990s." The meeting report, called Declaration of Talloires, suggested that national and international bodies set several targets to be achieved by 2000, among other things, the global eradication of polio.[5] Unfortunately, The Task Force missed identifying measles eradication as another equally worthy target.

WHO, as the undisputed world leader in disease prevention and control, particularly through public health, had to move fast and the Resolution was drafted and presented in the World Health Assembly (WHA) on 13 May 1988. Resolution 41.28 was passed unanimously.[6]

The Resolution: WHA 41.28

The Resolution declared, *"the commitment of WHO to the global eradication of poliomyelitis by the year 2000."*[6] *The Resolution emphasized "that eradication efforts should be pursued in ways which strengthened the development of the Expaned Programme on Immunisation as a whole, fostering its contribution, in turn, to the development of the health infrastructure and of primary health care."*

The message was clear: polio eradication, necessarily vertical, should be balanced by helping the development of health infrastructure and primary healthcare. What is the health infrastructure? Medicine -- modern, science-supported medicine -- consists of public health, healthcare and research. Public health is for disease control for which public health surveillance of all relevant diseases was essential; healthcare with adequate laboratory diagnostic support for quality service is to fulfill the felt need of all people; research is to keep raising their bars constantly.

Public health does not tolerate infectious diseases that can be prevented in individuals and controlled in the community. EPI had targeted six childhood diseases for prevention and control. Expanding and establishing universal primary healthcare and public health infrastructure were the natural lines of its growth, if so desired, if so designed. The health infrastructure of the polio eradicated world should be a lot better than that of the pre-eradication world. That was the spirit explicit in the Resolution.

The Resolution cited the *"the goal endorsed by the Thirtieth World Health Assembly in 1977 (resolution WHA 30.53) – the provision of immunization for all children of the world by 1990 – that will lead to further marked reductions in the incidence of most of the target diseases."*

It recognized: *"that the global eradication of poliomyelitis by the year 2000 represents both a fitting challenge to be undertaken now, on the Organization's fortieth anniversary, and an appropriate gift, together with the eradication of smallpox, from the twentieth to the twenty-first century."*

The desire was that the achievement of the global polio eradication goal *"will be facilitated by the continued strengthening of the Expanded Programme on Immunisation within the context of primary healthcare and by improving current poliomyelitis vaccines and clinical and laboratory surveillance."* [6]

Deja vu: during the middle of the smallpox eradication program, the smallpox vaccine was improved – with a better vaccine, freeze-dried, and a better vaccination tool, the bifurcated needle. Of the two polio vaccines, IPV had already been improved to near-perfection by Dutch and French scientists. OPV was not amenable to improvement. So, what was intended by the phrase *"by improving current vaccines"*?

Was it a reminder that OPV was not a good vaccine? The availability of 'vaccines', not just one 'vaccine', had been noted in the Resolution. That was in spite of the EPI policy of the exclusive use of only one vaccine, namely OPV. The Resolution recognized that there were *vaccines* to be used appropriately. Vaccines against polio are IPV and OPV.

EPI had failed to incorporate any disease surveillance in its purview, and the one proposed simple but efficient model was not endorsed.[6,7] That model consisted of all doctors, both in the government clinics and hospitals and in private clinics and hospitals reporting all cases of the target diseases of EPI, and important and outbreak-prone infectious diseases not targeted under EPI – in children and in adults. The system was at district level, so that the turn around time for any necessary investigations and disease control interventions was just a day or two. The disease reporting was kept very simple, without the need to fill out any elaborate forms. Being modular, district as the unit, it could be replicated at will, covering the whole country in a short time. It was extremely inexpensive too.[7,8] Without surveillance of even the target diseases of EPI, it remains a vertical vaccine-delivery platform even now.[4]

All-disease surveillance system that included polio was not promoted. So, vertical 'one-disease' surveillance had to be designed for polio eradication – the opportunity to strengthen EPI with broader multi-disease surveillance and to promote primary healthcare built around EPI, was sadly missed.

The Resolution had requested the Director-General of WHO to: *"strengthen planning, training and supervision within national immunisation programmes and undertaking country-specific evaluation to take corrective action towards achieving the goal of eradication in countries with coverage of less than 70%"* Had the Director-General acted upon this one special request, in the three Regions in need, we believe polio could have been eradicated globally by the target year of 2000 or latest within a few more years.

The call included *"strengthening clinical laboratory services"* in countries that lacked them. What was eventually done instead was to create stand-alone polio laboratories under WHO supervision – another vertical project. Even today, many district hospitals in India, each catering to the secondary healthcare needs of 2-3 million people, do not have any microbiology department to fulfill the requirements of clinical laboratory services.[9]

The resolution had requested the WHO Director-General *"to submit regular plans and reports of progress concerning the poliomyelitis eradication effort through the Executive Board to the Health Assembly, in the context of progress to be achieved by the Expanded Programme on Immunisation."* This shows that the World Health Assembly assumed the role as the apex agency in charge of eradication; its Executive Board to keep watch on the program; and WHO Director-General to function as the 'War General' of the war on polio.

Was not this design unwise and flawed in principle? A country's president may be the civilian top or supreme commander of its armed forces – but the president should not act as the War General. Similarly, the Director General is the top official of WHO but should not function as the War General which by itself is a full time professional job. The War General had to be answerable and accountable to the World Health Assembly through the WHO Director General. Did not the design (that we consider unwise) deprive the WHA of objectivity, by assigning to itself the responsibility for execution of the eradication program?

There existed sufficient knowledge to ensure polio eradication using the already available vaccines. We are 100% sure. When we read the Resolution as one entity, the target set for 2000, with 12 years to the finishing line, it seems to tell us that the experts who drafted it considered eradication achievable with the existing vaccines, perhaps with minor improvements if found necessary. Was such optimism and confidence of success the reason behind this design for WHA to be the apex agency?

There were, already, models of polio elimination with complete success in Scandinavian countries, providing proof of principle and sure-fire strategy for global eradication. Did not the drafters of the Resolution know about them? We are quite sure they did.

What was the endpoint of polio eradication, the finishing line? For smallpox eradication, the endpoint was zero case of smallpox. There were two virus variants causing smallpox, with their formal names as *Variola major* and *Alastrim* (or *Variola minor*) – both were eradicated using vaccinia virus vaccine, popularly known as smallpox vaccine.

Similarly, there were two virus variants causing polio – wild polioviruses and Sabin vaccine polioviruses in OPV. Wild viruses caused the natural disease of polio. Sabin vaccine viruses caused polio, clinically indistinguishable from natural polio. Wild and vaccine viruses came as three separate antigenic types or serotypes, 1, 2 and 3 – so altogether six viruses. Vaccine viruses caused polio only in countries using OPV. If you target both for eradication, IPV was the tool. Countries using IPV had no natural polio or vaccine-virus polio. OPV could, theoretically, eradicate wild virus polio, but not vaccine-virus polio. Was not the endpoint of eradication zero polio due to any of the six viruses? If polio case count had to be zero, all polioviruses had to be eliminated from transmission. So, the endpoint of polio eradication, to be achieved by the year 2000, had to be zero case of polio, in which case OPV was incompatible with polio eradication.

When zero smallpox was reached, automatically virus transmission had stopped. In non-immune persons, the case-to-infection ratio of smallpox was nearly one. That meant that nearly every case of infection manifested as disease – silent transmission was not a problem. If no case occurred within the equivalent interval of one incubation period of smallpox, after the previous case, that meant no more transmission -- no smallpox disease meant no smallpox virus transmission.

Polio is not that simple: the case-to-infection ratio of wild polioviruses is 1/200-2000: one paralytic case for 200-2000 non-immune children infected. If surveillance is good and sufficiently long-term, polio cases would surely show up as acute flaccid paralysis (AFP), if the transmission was continuing. Like the crocodile-infested waters -- watch for sufficient time, and some snout will show up. No snout for one minute does not mean no crocodile – only no snout after sufficient time of watching would mean no crocodile.

By definition, eradication is zero transmission of the agent – here, the six polioviruses.[10] The case-to-infection ratio of vaccine viruses is orders of magnitude lower than that of wild viruses. So it was going to be tricky to prove the absence of silent transmission of vaccine viruses. So it was of critical importance that we stopped feeding children with OPV as early as possible. If the target was the year 2000, OPV should have been ramped down, and IPV ramped up to ensure that no OPV was given to children some time before 2000. That should have been part of the strategy and tactics of polio eradication by 2000.

Global polio eradication program had to create circumstances to achieve that target and that endpoint. Introduction and incremental immunization coverage with IPV was that common sense circumstance. The timing had to be planned in the war room. If the war had to be won by the year 2000, and now we were in 1988, when would you suggest we introduce IPV and when would you want all OPV stopped? We argue that the program had to discontinue all OPV some reasonable time before 2000, the target year of eradication.

The Resolution did not spell out any endpoint, but there was no need – eradication subsumed all polio caused by any poliovirus. That is our interpretation. Unfortunately, the polio eradication program experts did not apparently read this correctly – they believed only wild virus polio was to be eradicated. That was another very disturbing turn of events. Here was the critical importance of the need for cool objectivity without the fog of subjectivity.

What was its result? During the course of the eradication program, its leaders classified vaccine-polio, called 'vaccine-associated paralytic polio', VAPP, in the vaccinated children as well as in their contacts, as "non-polio acute flaccid paralysis". The most likely reason for this was that it was at once both adverse reaction to OPV as well as polio. Subjectively the OPV-protagonists saw VAPP as adverse reaction to OPV, whereas any third party, with objectivity, would have seen it as no less polio than natural polio.

Yes, that is right: the program did not count VAPP as polio in OPV-using countries as it was, by their definition, non-polio. We do not quite know how this idea crept into the interpretation of the Resolution – we submit that it went against its letter and spirit.

In a lighter vein -- *"When I use a word, it means just what I choose it to mean – neither more, nor less"* said Humpty Dumpty in Lewis Carroll's Alice in Wonderland. When we say Lewis Carroll, we mean Charles Lutwidge Dodgson, the eccentric mathematician-logician who used the pen name, Lewis Carroll.

Socrates is credited as saying: "The best possible way to speak consists in using names all (or most) of which are like the things they name (that is, are appropriate to them), while the worst is to use the opposite kind of names."[11] Back to serious issues. VAPP by definition is polio, paralytic polio to be clear, caused by vaccine virus. No doubt about it. It is definitely not non-polio acute flaccid paralysis (AFP).

Who was supposed to be responsible for achieving the goal of eradication? Member states were urged to: *"to intensify surveillance to ensure prompt identification and investigation of cases of poliomyelitis and control of outbreaks and accurate and timely reporting of cases at national and international levels".* There was hardly a surveillance component in EPI – and there was no design either. Yet, countries were being urged to intensify surveillance. Intensify without first establishing surveillance?

EPI in most countries in the three relevant Regions – SE Asia, Africa and Eastern Mediterranean – was still an under-performing vaccine delivery platform and not a disease control program. Was the ball in the courts of such countries to do everything the Resolution demanded?

Was EPI in those countries supposed to go from polio endemic state, bypass polio 'control' and go straight for 'elimination' so that global eradication may succeed? Should not the creation of a platform of polio 'control' be the take-off runway of eradication?

The Resolution was passed unanimously: goal achieved? Was the Resolution mistakenly taken as the goal and were the countries themselves expected to eliminate polio in the countries that voted to pass the Resolution through their EPI? The follow-up actions and responses to the Resolution were relaxed. Now, was the job in each country EPI's purview?

Formidable obstacles in the three Regions

As pointed out earlier, the 1988 Resolution had recognized that: *"regional eradication goals by or before the year 2000 have already been set in in the Regions of the Americas, Europe and the Western Pacific".* Therefore, the Resolution was, in fact, asking WHO to essentially extend the geographic extent of polio elimination to the three Regions of SE Asia, Africa and Eastern Mediterranean from the Regions of Americas, Europe and Western Pacific, so as to cover the whole world.

The obvious and immediate responsibility of WHO was in the three Regions of SE Asia, Africa and the Eastern Mediterranean, to control polio and graduate to elimination – to design tactics, to work with each country government, to help improve EPI coverage, to progressively control polio and reach elimination. The three Regions have Regional Offices, just like the Regions of the Americas, Europe and the Western Pacific. Why were roles and responsibilities not copied from these Regions and transplanted in the three needy Regions?

The spirit of the clauses in the Resolution had clearly identified the need for targeted research to troubleshoot and problem-solve. Such research required careful planning. Unfortunately, research even into the efficacy and safety of OPV and IPV in different geographic settings was not designed on time. The two available vaccines were not evaluated and compared for their pluses and minuses. We attempt to compare the vaccines in the next chapter.

Many countries in the Regions of SE Asia, Africa and the Eastern Mediterranean had two major obstacles as far as OPV was concerned. The low coverage (<70%) was already recognized in the Resolution – "failure to vaccinate". Widely known, but not spelt out, was the other problem of low vaccine efficacy – "failure of vaccine". The third problem was the occurrence of VAPP, due to the vaccine.

The Resolution said [6]: *"[WHO] encourages Member States which have not yet attained a 70% coverage rate to accelerate their efforts so as to surpass this level as quickly as possible through means which also improve and sustain the coverage for the other vaccines included within the national immunization programmes."*

Wishes are not horses. As polioviruses are highly contagious, the required coverage would have been better than 95%. How could that be achieved from the starting point of less than 70% coverage?

The problem of low OPV efficacy was staring at WHO and EPI right from the year of inception of EPI, in 1974. Too many 'vaccine-failure' cases of WPV polio were occurring in many countries in these three Regions. Did they ever get counted? Because of the high frequency of vaccine failure cases of WPV polio, the benchmark of 95% coverage was not just for 3 doses, but a sufficient number of doses that would translate to near-100% protective efficacy against WPV polio. The number of doses had to be determined by studies and titrated for each country with vaccine failure polio. Such studies had to be started in 1988. Unfortunately they were not done.

The Resolution had requested the WHO Director-General to act on: *"Strengthening, planning, training and supervision within national immunization programmes and undertaking country-specific evaluation to facilitate corrective action towards achieving the goal of eradication in countries with coverage of less than 70%."* If quick action had been initiated on this clause, the very low vaccine efficacy in many countries could have been detected very early and corrective actions taken in order to keep the time line of eradication by 2000. The wages of neglect is failure.

Since eradication means no vaccine-failure polio as well as vaccine-caused polio – all polio had to be accepted as vaccine-preventable if vaccine choice was made correctly. The Regions of Europe, Western Pacific and the Americas had many countries using IPV; they had no vaccine failure polio or vaccine-caused polio. Other countries that were using OPV had problems of vaccine failure and vaccine-caused polio. The lessons were quite clear if the vision was objective and unbiased.

So, the models of the Americas, Europe and the Western Pacific were not quite adequate for eradication as long as some countries were still using OPV. The eradication program had its jobs cut out: in these well-performing

Regions, to replace OPV with IPV and in the three poor-performing Regions to strengthen the health infrastructure and EPI and also to plan to follow in the footsteps of the well-performing Regions.

Instead of designing suitable tactics and logistics in each of the six Regions – as the immediate top priority of WHO -- the simplistic idea of one size must fit all was applied.

Americas Region was certified WPV-eradicated in 1994, 3 years after their last case in 1991. Western Pacific Region was so certified in 2000, 3 years after their last case in 1997. European Region was certified in 2002, 3 years after their last case in 1998. Subsequently, many countries in these 3 Regions have replaced OPV with IPV on their own, in spite of the fact the global program had not demanded that.

However, no Region has yet fully eradicated all polio, which remains an embarrassing reality for the eradication program even in 2020.

Why were three Regions lagging behind?

The contrast between the three relatively well-performing and the three poorly performing Regions had to be understood if corrective actions were to be designed. What were the important reasons why the latter Regions lagged? We are not aware of any attempt on the part of WHO or the eradication program to have explored the reasons. In medicine, any malady should be diagnosed first and only then its remedy can be determined and applied. A diagnosis must precede therapy.

OPV, performing reasonably well in the three former Regions was not satisfactorily efficacious in many countries in the three latter Regions. OPV is an oral vaccine. Live attenuated oral typhoid vaccine Ty21A did well in the Americas Region but performed worse in the Eastern Mediterranean Region (EMR). Rotavirus vaccine that did well in the Americas did not do so in Africa Region.[23] Thus; orally given live vaccines did poorly in many countries of the three latter Regions. This was first demonstrated in relation to OPV, by a WHO-sponsored study, way back in 1968-69, in one country in the SEA Region.[13]

Did WHO experts worry about it, develop a hypothesis why, or develop a strategy to improve upon vaccine efficacy? Or at least realistically plan to introduce the better vaccine IPV? No, they did not, but the problem was simply swept under the carpet.

For polio, we have two vaccines – OPV, not very efficacious and IPV that was exquisitely efficacious. IPV had been shown to have extremely high vaccine efficacy in the limited studies that had been done over the years in different settings in countries of the Regions of SE Asia, Africa and EMR. The spirit and letter of the Resolution was global eradication of polio. OPV had to be ramped down, and IPV ramped up. The setting of time for these steps was the job of the war room planners. Failing to plan is planning to fail.

How well was modern medicine adopted in the three Regions?

We know India well. Modern medicine was transplanted in India only a little more than 100 years ago 25.[14] So also in China. While the transplant has taken somewhat better in China, it has not been so, in India. Both OPV and IPV are manufactured in China, OPV from the 1960s and IPV rather recently, but neither vaccine is yet made in India. Instead, vaccines are imported as bulk concentrates and diluted and filled in vials as finished products. China has made IPV by inactivating Sabin strains of polioviruses and will soon be using it to replace OPV. A Chinese scientist was awarded the Nobel Prize in Medicine for malaria research conducted under the government's auspices – that resulted in developing Artimesenin. These are just to illustrate the different mindsets of the peoples and leaders of many nations into which modern medicine was transplanted.

Experts in epidemiology and public health from cultures that had inherited, not transplanted, modern medicine, had probably taken modern medicine as granted and not fully grasped the cultural issues impinging on polio eradication. All countries were not in the same boat. The more important contrast is the presence of vibrant public health infrastructure in China, Sri Lanka and Thailand, while India and many others in the three Regions we named above, do not have even a public health department in the national government. Therefore India was compelled to have vertical programs – against TB, malaria, even polio. India's polio eradication program was a vertical one, not nested in EPI, which itself is another vertical program not nested either in public health or in universal healthcare.

This is just to illustrate that the traditional and deep-rooted cultures in many countries of the three Regions in need of help in polio eradication have, philosophical, sociological, anthropological and cultural differences that have stood in the way of absorbing modern medicine – public health, universal healthcare and research – into their ethos. We are not experts in this area – but our point is that this contrast had to be explored by WHO in order to understand why EPI was not performing well – also if polio could be eliminated through EPI.

Here, a country by country approach was absolutely necessary – absolutely not one size must fit all approach. EPI is a win for children, win for parents and families, win for the national economy, and win for vaccine manufacturers. Win-win-win-win and yet EPI remains in need of repair? If that was not understood, how could we rely on countries to eradicate polio through EPI?

Thomas Abraham in his book, "Polio. The Odyssey of Eradication" quotes a Nigerian asking him: *"Why this polio,*

polio, when the parents had many unmet healthcare needs for their children? "[15] Polio eradication had to be nested within the context of providing for people's urgent and unmet needs of healthcare.

Food culture in the three Regions

As one travels around, the standards of food hygiene will appear quite different in the different countries of different Regions. Travel westward from Europe -- people in most countries in Europe and the Americas use spoon, knives and forks to eat with. Food safety is taken very seriously. Reach Japan, China, and Viet Nam and travel westward: people in Western Pacific Region countries use chopsticks, spoons or forks to put food in the mouth. They do not serve food with bare hands. They enforce and practice food hygiene.

Come to the Indian subcontinent – Bangladesh, Nepal, India, Pakistan – people serve food and eat with hands and fingers. Right through the Middle East to the north and Africa to the south, people in many countries eat using hands and fingers. For many, cleanliness is visual and aesthetic, not microbiological.

In short, in several countries in the 3 Regions, food hygiene is quite bad, keeping food uncovered in the open, serving with bare hands and eating also with bare hands. Countries in these Regions have more diarrheal diseases, dysenteries, typhoid fever, cholera, faecal-oral transmitted hepatitis A and E and so on.

What does poor food hygiene got to do with the performance of OPV? The problems with low efficacy of oral vaccines seemed to go parallel with low food hygiene and repeated gastrointestinal infections and diarrheal diseases. It is generally in those countries in which general sanitation and particularly food hygiene are poor that children do not get infected by vaccine polioviruses as readily as in countries with high standards of sanitation and food hygiene. The two phenomena seem to be related – but how?

Tropical and subtropical developing countries are the ones with both these two phenomena. Yet, such countries do not have any advantage against wild polioviruses.

So we need to explain the puzzle – that of easy and early infection by wild viruses while vaccine viruses are resisted from infection of the gut. In Chapter 6 we suggest that the reason why wild viruses catch children young but OPV fails to infect them could be because of two different routes of entry into the body – wild viruses by the nose and vaccine viruses by the mouth. That explains only why wild and vaccine viruses behave differently, but not why vaccine viruses do not readily infect the guts of children.

There is a stage of immunity called innate immunity. Effective immunity consists of innate immunity, reacting to any invading microbe or inoculated antigen immediately, and adaptive immunity which takes time to develop. The function of innate immunity is to first recognize the entry of a microbe in the forbidden territories of the body, to distinguish between harmless microbes that could be ignored and potentially disease-causing microbes to be dealt with severely. While wild polioviruses are to be fought with adaptive immunity, vaccine polioviruses are much weakened (attenuated) and may be ignored. In guts without challenges from many microbes, the innate immunity responds readily even to the vaccine viruses. In guts which are always fighting against many nasty microbes, the vaccine viruses are recognized as non-threatening and ignored without detriment. Let us say the innate immunity is extra-ready to do its job of discriminating between virulent polioviruses and attenuated polioviruses. This explanation is not proven but merely proposed as plausible, especially for want of any other proven explanation.

If both EPI and polio eradication were of equal priority for WHO, the only way to go forward was to include IPV through EPI and top up with OPV through campaigns only where and when needed. IPV was EPI-friendly as only 2 or 3 doses were enough. So the choice of vaccine, OPV or IPV was not a simple choice between two vaccines, but between eradication through EPI or eradication bypassing the EPI system.[16,17]

Summation

The WHA resolution gave WHO twelve years to implement the necessary interventions and monitoring for polio eradication, and bring polio down to zero, essentially in the three WHO Regions of Africa, Eastern Mediterranean and South-East Asia. As the Resolution itself was drafted by WHO officials, the target year of 2000 was actually self-imposed but realistic. The Regions of the Americas, Western Pacific and Europe did not need any guidance or expertise from WHO except for planning the early transition from OPV to IPV. However, the planning of strategy and tactics in the three needy Regions were very complex and had to be carefully designed in the program's war room. We have no information that there was a proper war room for the war that was declared in 1988.

The Resolution does not seem to have been diligently followed in letter and spirit. The two symposia on eradication strategy and tactics organized by independent agencies in 1993 in Jerusalem and 2000 in Paris, described in Chapter 6, were not apparently taken seriously by the global polio eradication program. The program itself does not seem to have organised such critical review meetings at any times to see how far the interventions and monitoring followed the stipulations of the Resolution.

The WHA Resolution for global polio eradication was binding on WHO and all member countries, since WHA is the assembly of Ministers of Health from all countries. The delay of two decades and yet the shore not sighted for landing, is clearly the result of faulty plans of actions and consequent failure to reach the goal. This malady must be remedied but diagnosis must precede treatment. The diagnosis is the purpose of this book. We will also go further and offer prescriptions for curing the malady.

§§§

2. INTRODUCTION TO THE WEAPONS OF WAR

The War General must choose the right weapons at the right time to win the war and to minimise collateral damage. The longer the war, the higher the collateral damage.

The war simile for polio eradication is appropriate for many reasons. It highlights the urgency and seriousness of purpose. The enemy is poliovirus – actually polioviruses, as there are three distinct antigenic types (or serotypes), identified as 1, 2 and 3. Polio eradication has strategy, tactics and logistics, terms borrowed from war parlance. Therefore vaccines against polio are like weapons of war.

The war simile ends here. This war has no violence. Vaccines against polio do not draw blood. As mentioned earlier, there are two vaccines, IPV and OPV. There are two chapters that describe them in greater detail and depth, chapters 4 and 5. What a vaccine does is to render the vaccinated child protected from the target disease. Protection is afforded by immunity. Immunity is an individual's attribute. The immune child is ordinarily not protected from poliovirus infection when exposed but is protected from paralytic disease even when infected.

Polioviruses are contagious – spreading person to person. The infected person, child or grown-up, sheds the virus into the environment, putting others at risk of catching the infection. If the newly infected was not immune, he/she would shed lots of viruses, whether or not he/she develops the disease. If the newly infected person was immune, he/she would shed far less virus – in quantum and duration. Therefore the probability of new infection in non-immune children declines. Thus, in a community in which a large proportion are vaccinated, hence immune, the number of new infections are reduced, creating a spiral of less new infections and less disease burden.

If such immunity pressure is sustained in the community, the infection dies out in that community. The cumulative effect of sustained immunization is the steady decline in disease burden and infection burden until the infection disappears altogether. This is the principle of elimination of infection in a country that has sustained high immunization coverage. When all countries achieve elimination, the infection will be globally eradicated.

All these are strictly contingent upon the vaccine being highly efficacious in immunising the vaccinated children. Although many use the terms vaccination and immunization interchangeably, as if synonymous, a vaccine with low efficacy will not immunise all vaccinated children. So, the intended result of immunization, rendering the child immune, depends on the efficacy of the vaccine. Vaccination with a limited number of doses of a vaccine of low efficacy is only a ritual without full benefit. A sharp axe will cut the tree in a few strokes, but a blunt axe will need many more strokes -- same with highly efficacious vaccine and poorly efficacious vaccine.

Since immunity is needed before the child is exposed to infection, the poorly efficacious vaccine may fail to immunise the child when it was needed. In that case, the poorly efficacious vaccine will not slow down the cycle of infection, in other words, the circulation of the target virus, in the community. That will prolong the control program. In the war against polio, the weapon's quality is crucial.

IPV, inactivated poliovirus vaccine

IPV was the first of the two vaccines, licensed in USA, Canada and Scandinavian countries in 1955. Its production procedure was improved upon the earlier process in the early 1980s in the Netherlands and France. At that time it was called IPV of enhanced potency or eIPV, but by the end of 1980s, all IPV was eIPV. Since then, when we say IPV, we mean the modified high potency IPV. The new process also resulted in a lower cost of vaccine production than the earlier version. However, the vaccine price is determined not by production cost alone but also by demand, the margin of profit, competition etc.

IPV was excluded from EPI, and the only demand for IPV was in rich countries. Therefore the volume turnover remained low and price of the vaccine became high. IPV was also excluded from the global polio eradication program – further affecting the future of vaccine market. Thus the demand and projected future demand remained relatively small. Only very few manufacturers survived in the market; all others closed shop. Thus IPV became a seller's vaccine, not a buyer's vaccine. The price became too high for low and middle-income countries to afford it. The high price further reduced the demand – further pushing the price up. In short, unwise policies made by the global public health leaders in effect resulted in making IPV out of reach of low-income countries.

IPV is inoculated by injection. Two doses given 4 to 6 months apart with the first dose at or after 14 weeks of age will induce immunity in virtually all children, and that immunity is long-lived also. One additional dose, usually called booster dose, given at a convenient time, in the second year of life or fifth year of life, will boost immunity to very high levels and will ensure life-long immunity. IPV can be combined with other injectable vaccine antigens. The most popular combination vaccine has six components, hence called hexavalent – diphtheria, tetanus, pertussis, hepatitis B and *Haemophilus influenzae* type b antigens plus IPV. The hexavalent vaccine can fit into the conventional schedule of 3 doses at 6, 10, and 14 weeks of age and one booster dose in the second year of life. As IPV itself has three separate antigens of poliovirus types 1, 2 and 3, the 6 component vaccine actually has eight components. That is a matter of detail – the vaccine is known as hexavalent.

OPV, oral polio vaccine

Oral polio vaccine contains live attenuated polioviruses. The dictionary meaning of attenuation is to weaken – hence the expression weakened polioviruses is commonly used.

Natural polioviruses, also called wild polioviruses, infect only humans under natural conditions. Infection, broadly speaking, results in three events in all infected persons:
- Invasion and multiplication in body tissues and organs
- Shedding of viruses so as to infect others and to perpetuate virus survival
- Development of immunity

In a small minority of individuals infected with poliovirus, a pathology (disease of body tissue/organs) develops as a consequence of invasion and multiplication of the virus. Poliovirus pathology is in the spinal cord, with the resulting muscle paralysis due to lost innervation.

We saw that IPV does not infect – hence no virus multiplication, no shedding, no pathology, just immunity alone. OPV is infectious, but it may not infect everyone who swallows it. If a person is infected, the same three evets follow: invasion/multiplication, virus shedding and development of immunity. Just very rarely, far more infrequently than in the case of natural/wild poliovirus, the virus may invade the spinal cord and cause pathology and muscle paralysis – the illness is called 'vaccine-associated paralytic polio' (VAPP). Attenuation is the removal of the disease potential – otherwise known as virulence. For poliovirus, it is 'neurovirulence'. Obviously, attenuation is incomplete in OPV.

Attenuation was through careful laboratory manipulation of wild polioviruses until they lost the ability to cause pathology in the spinal cords of monkeys when they were directly injected into the spinal cord. These complicated steps were carefully done by the famous bio-scientist, Albert Sabin, working in Cincinnati, USA. Sabin attenuated all three poliovirus types – the resultant viruses were called 'vaccine strains' or 'Sabin strains'.

OPV could be trivalent (containing types 1, 2 and 3) or monovalent (type 1, 2 or 3) or bivalent (types 1 and 3).

OPV was first licensed in the USA in 1961, and thereafter it became more popular than IPV; in 1964 USA policy shifted from IPV to OPV; from 1968, no IPV was available in the USA.

Eventually, the USA switched back to exclusive use of IPV in the year 1999. The reason for that switch was the problem of VAPP – averages of 8-10 children were developing VAPP annually from 1962, until 1999. OPV is not completely safe; safety problem is more severe in children with certain forms of immune deficiency. Note the timing – 2000 was the target year for global polio eradication; USA could not have made the grade with VAPP occurring every year.

We saw how important efficacy is for a vaccine. OPV has a problem with efficacy – its efficacy is not uniform universally. IPV has very high efficacy in all countries, but OPV has a wide range of efficacy – excellent in rich countries, somewhat less in some countries and very low in many low-income countries, especially in the tropics and sub-tropics.

Where efficacy is low, children need repeated doses, 10-20 or even more – for which campaigns are essential – even house-to-house campaigns are needed to reach all children multiple times.

Don't blame the weapons for not winning the war

The war has not been won even as we write this in 2020, thirty-two years since the start. The reasons are not difficult to determine – they are not even complicated but quite simple.

The polio eradicators, guided by WHO, chose one of the two weapons for exclusive use, from the start in 1988 till 2016.

Even then, the second weapon was used in a rationed and gingerly manner, as we shall see elaborated in chapters to follow. However, the exclusive use of OPV can be singled out and proved to be the reason for not winning the war on polio.

Surely OPV had an important role in the war, but its role had to be tactically positioned in the grand strategy of the war, in the short, medium and long terms – all in 12 years, from 1988 to 2000. The tactical positioning of IPV, the incomparably more powerful weapon than OPV, was unavoidable if the war had to be won in 12 years, or, plus a few more years if found necessary. But 20 more years and no victory in sight is not a simple matter of minor mishap, but an instance of gross public health negligence.

The potter has every right to break his creation, however beautiful and intricate. But if the potter's creation was paid for, and morally belonged to the payer, the potter has no right to break it before delivery.

There is a concept called accountability. We believe that the polio eradicators are accountable to the world for the predicament the world is facing with the war on polio not yet won.

Summation

The war on polio was declared with confidence that the available weapons were sufficient to defeat the enemy and win the war. Fortunately, the attackers had two vaccines which were potentially a great asset. Unfortunately, the attackers misread the confidence of the drafters of the WHA Resolution on polio eradication described in the first chapter. Instead of the confidence of resolution drafters, the attackers had over-confidence amounting to unjustified hubris in one of the two weapons.

§§§

3. AN INSTRUMENT TO COMPARE VACCINES, OPV AND IPV

"Choices are the hinges of destiny" Edwin Markham

The two vaccines against polio, IPV and OPV, have many contrasting properties and could be used singly or in combination formats. Neither vaccine was patented by the USA scientists who developed it – Jonas Salk (IPV) or Albert Sabin (OPV). IPV was licensed in the USA in 1955 and monovalent type 1 OPV in 1961 and trivalent OPV in 1964. A lot of debate about the characteristics and usefulness of the two vaccines – controversies actually -- had also followed their licensing in the USA. All other vaccines developed in the second half of the twentieth century have been patented, and the companies behind them were interested in promoting their vaccines.

When looked at the issue objectively, dispassionately and unemotionally, it becomes clear that perhaps the controversies were more personality-based – Sabin versus Salk – than science-based.

As IPV was not patented, no company was particularly interested in promoting it, except those who manufactured and marketed it. The agency that spearheaded its development, the National Foundation for Infantile Paralysis (described in chapters to follow), gradually withdrew from the scene having accomplished its mission of gifting a vaccine to the world. Because IPV was abandoned in the USA after OPV became popular, no US company remained interested in manufacturing it – only European companies did. The demand for IPV was then limited to a few European nations and a few Canadian Provinces not involved in the rather irrational controversies.

Unlike Salk, Sabin himself had actively promoted the manufacture of OPV in many countries, personally visiting and training scientists and also providing seed viruses – thus Russia, China, Iran, Vietnam, Indonesia, India, Brazil and Mexico had established OPV production in the 1960s and 1970s, mostly in the government sector. The government in India had ordered the discontinuation of OPV manufacture (in the semi-private institution that Sabin had himself chosen as the ideal place for establishing the vaccine unit), in 1974, as a result of what we believe was bureaucratic bungling. All other countries continued to be self-sufficient for OPV and Brazil and Indonesia earned much foreign exchange by exporting OPV to many countries, including India.

Sabin donated his entire remaining stock of seed virus strains to the WHO in 1972 after which WHO assumed 'custodianship' of Sabin's vaccine virus strains, and the next year constituted a Consultative Group in which Sabin was a member, but not Salk[1].

Thereafter WHO promoted OPV, ensuring vaccine quality of various producers. In 1974 WHO included only OPV in EPI, not IPV. IPV had no patronage. Policymakers in developing countries and even many global public health opinion leaders seem to have misunderstood the fact of OPV promotion by WHO to mean that IPV was unsuitable in national immunization programmes, or, at least that IPV was inferior to OPV.

Our purpose here is to set objective criteria to compare and contrast the pluses and minuses of the two vaccines and to apply them for such comparison. We are not aware of such an exercise done ever before, in spite of its importance and value in policy design in public health, particularly in polio eradication.

A vaccine's MEF is to safely protect the vaccinated child

MEF is the *minimum essential function* – that which makes a vaccine a good vaccine. A vaccine is given to children when they are well – hence,

(a) it should be *safe* from serious adverse effect (or serious adverse reaction) and

(b) it should protect them from the target disease with high probability after the recommended number of doses – 2, 3, 4 or 5 – in other words it should be *efficacious*.

Under the WHO Expanded Program on Immunization (EPI) there is a system of monitoring 'adverse events following immunization' (AEFI). Disease events occurring within a reasonable period of any immunization are included in AEFI, irrespective of its causal relationship with immunization. Every episode of AEFI must be investigated to determine if the adverse event was causally associated with the vaccination that preceded it. Most disease events during the post-vaccination period, as in any other similar time period, would be unrelated to immunization, in other words natural illnesses that would have occurred even if the vaccine had not been given. But that needs to be established, based on objective causality assessment. When the AEFI is an illness caused by the preceding vaccine dose, it is an adverse reaction to the vaccine, for the purpose of our context here.

'Serious adverse reaction' (serious AEFI), is an illness that requires hospitalization, or an illness that causes prolonged (chronic) symptoms/disability, or an illness that results in death -- caused by the vaccine and not merely coincidental. Fortunately, all approved vaccines are known for their safety from serious adverse reactions, except one -- OPV.

Efficacy is a quality that can be quantified with the metric of the immunising effect of vaccination, which results in protection against, or prevention of, disease in the vaccinated – the very reason why a vaccine is needed and is given. If 100 children are vaccinated and later exposed to infection by the disease-agent, how many will be protected from disease? Ideally, all vaccinated should be protected when efficacy would be 100%. If only half are protected, we may attribute an efficacy score of 50%.

In the case of most viral vaccines, the antibody response is a valid surrogate for clinical protection. In such cases, antibody has been shown to correlate with protection consistently. For such vaccines, for example, OPV and IPV, seroconversion rate (proportion converting from antibody-negative to positive) is equal to vaccine efficacy.

Thus the two major qualities we seek in any vaccine, MEF in other words, are safety and efficacy of the vaccine. A safe vaccine is one that does not cause a serious adverse reaction. An efficacious vaccine is one with reasonably high efficacy score, ideally 100%, but in reality, it maybe 80-85% or more – even 70-75% or more. The higher the efficacy score, the better.

MEF scoring system for OPV, IPV

A simple but logical MEF score could be devised with 1 to 4 marks for safety and 1 to 4 marks for efficacy – the product of the two sets of marks could be the MEF score of a vaccine. Imagine we have two alternative vaccines against one disease. Once MEF is very favourable with a score of 4X4 =

16 for both vaccines, other qualities of vaccines such as cost, ease of administration, frequency of non-serious adverse effects etc. are helpful in vaccine choice, if one is faced with such a choice between two vaccines against one disease – like OPV and IPV.

If MEF score is unfavourable for one vaccine, then the decision to use such a vaccine must be very carefully considered. If the problem is with regards to safety, then ethics must guide a decision. If the problem is with efficacy, then ways must be designed to improve it. If the other vaccine has a favourable score, obviously that should be preferred.

If a vaccine with suboptimal MEF score has some other qualities in favour, then a decision to use it needs a careful appraisal. If the problem is with regards to safety, then a careful benefit-risk assessment is necessary. The risk of disease, by way of how common and how serious – reflecting the reverse, namely the benefit expected from vaccination, is one part of the equation. That must be weighed against the risk of serious adverse reaction from the vaccine itself – how common and how serious -- the other part of the equation. The benefit-risk assessment of the vaccine, if favourable, informs that the vaccine may have a role in a community level immunization program, in spite of low MEF score. We will return to these issues later on.

When WHO designed EPI and launched it in 1974, OPV was included in the list of EPI vaccines, and IPV excluded, apparently without a comparison of the two vaccines for safety and efficacy. Apparently, WHO experts had full familiarity with OPV but not with IPV. In 1972, the custodianship of OPV had been left in the hands of WHO. The next year Sabin was an invited member of the WHO Consultative Group on OPV. No provision was made for an option to even consider IPV. That was very strange, but not surprising. With expertise available and ownership established, OPV was a natural choice of WHO. The alternate hypothesis is that it was a copy from the then USA policy of the exclusive use of OPV. Were USA polio experts unduly influencing WHO policymakers? If the WHO policy was a copy of the USA policy, when the USA changed policy in 1999, to switch to IPV and abandon OPV, the WHO would have followed suit. It is reasonable to assume, therefore, that the WHO policy was independent of USA policy. It is reasonable to assume, under these circumstances, that WHO experts might have been biased and not even handed.

In our context regarding EPI, the WHO made a deliberate choice of the exclusive use of OPV, as if IPV had no role in EPI, although their MEF scores, as we present here, were not on par at all – the score that we will propose here, at first cut, will be based on the knowledge available in 1974, in order to assess how far that choice was justified in EPI. For that we will have to think back to 1974.

Later on we shall revisit the MEF scores and vaccine choice, appropriate for 1988 when global polio eradication was launched, and again for 2000-2001 when the eradication target year was missed – both with contemporaneously available information.

Vaccine safety assessment, as of 1974, when EPI was launched

IPV was universally safe from serious adverse reactions wherever it was used, and we give 4 marks for safety. There was a mishap in 1955, when IPV manufactured by one Cutter Company in the USA was faulty, as a result of which live virus was still present in the vaccine. The Cutter vaccine caused polio in a number of vaccinated children and it was removed from further use. That infamous episode is known as the Cutter Incident. The USA National Drugs Regulatory Agency made stringent quality control protocol and all IPV made ever since has been totally safe. The Cutter Incident is described in more details in the Chapter on IPV.

OPV caused, on rare occasions, but with measurable, hence predictable, frequency, a serious adverse reaction associated with a chronic disability or even death. True, it was of very low frequency, but, with very severe consequence when it occurred. It was clinically paralytic polio, indistinguishable from wild virus polio, the one the vaccine was supposed to protect against. The proportions of severe disease, extensive paralysis, even death, in children with vaccine-virus-induced polio are identical to those with polio caused by wild polioviruses. But the virus infecting such affected children was vaccine virus and not wild virus. This serious AEFI was named in the USA, as early as in 1964, as "vaccine-associated paralytic polio" (VAPP). WHO had, through its OPV Consultative Group, reconfirmed the occurrence of VAPP in European countries that were using OPV, and published its reports in 1976 and 1982. [2,3]

Strangely, not only the vaccinated child but a rare bystander (child or grown-up) in contact with the vaccinated child also got what was called VAPP. In the absence of vaccination, it is inaccurate to call it vaccine-associated; in reality, it is at best vaccine-virus-associated. But, what comes out of a vaccinated child cannot be equated to vaccine virus. So we have a semantic problem, reflecting a conceptual problem. The reasonable way to circumvent it is to name the virus Sabin strain of poliovirus. Alternatively, it could have been called "vaccine-derived poliovirus" – a name that was coined in 2001, as we will describe below. So polio in a contact of vaccinated child was caused by Sabin virus and not the vaccine virus.

Such polio was called, right or wrong, in the USA in 1964, "contact VAPP" as against "VAPP in the vaccinated". Contact VAPP was also described as early as in 1964, and could not have been ignored or justified according to moral and legal principles or even commonsense. But it was ignored and justified in the USA, even by experts, policymakers and Regulatory Agency – in the country that is otherwise a vehement and vocal critic of any human rights violation in any other country.

For these two reasons, VAPP in the vaccinated and so-called contact VAPP, we cannot give four marks for safety -- we could give 3 marks, considering the low frequency of VAPP. On the other hand, considering the severity of VAPP -- death in a few, and, life-long disability in survivors -- the safety score should be less than 3, such as 2. Shall we settle on a score of 2.5?

Knowing that OPV had safety problems, why was a disinterested appraisal not made before recommending it for universal and exclusive use by WHO? Why was the touchstone of biomedical ethics not applied in spite of the safety questions?

Paternalistic attitude on the part of the policymakers towards the general public, even in public health interventions, was the norm in the 1960s and 1970s. That changed only in the late 1980s towards a fair and humane attitude – due to the revised thinking on attitudes of policymakers in the context of AIDS, when human rights gained wide acceptance in medical and public health ethics. So, the late 1980s was a time when the ethics of the exclusive use of OPV should have been examined, both in the USA and in WHO.

Vaccine efficacy evaluation, as of 1974, when EPI was launched

By 1974 the very high vaccine efficacy of IPV was widely recognised in USA, Canada, Finland, Sweden and Norway, wherever IPV was used. Indeed, Sweden, Finland, Norway and Iceland had eliminated wild virus polio without risk of

VAPP within a few years of the exclusive use of IPV, foretelling the future possibility of polio eradication.

IPV was not available in developing countries; hence efficacy information was not documented. In developed countries, vaccine efficacy was virtually 100%, for a score of 4 marks. Unless proved otherwise the same would hold true for developing countries also – it was never ever proven otherwise.

By 1974, the very high vaccine efficacy of OPV (3 doses) was also widely recognised in USA, UK and a few European countries – where efficacy was virtually 100%, for a score of 4. No child had developed wild-virus polio after taking the three doses of OPV.

During the late 1960s, the world's first cases of polio in spite of 3 doses of OPV (vaccine-failure polio) were documented in Vellore.[4,5] The sub-optimal rate of antibody response to OPV, documented by WHO-funded studies during 1968-69, provided the reason for vaccine-failure polio cases. By 1974 it had been widely recognised that there was some serious problem with antibody response, hence vaccine efficacy, in children in tropical developing countries, to the orally fed OPV. In summary, the efficacy score of OPV in countries like India, Pakistan, Kenya, Nigeria etc. was not 4 but at best 3, as of 1974.

MEF scores of IPV and OPV as in 1974, when EPI was launched

The MEF score of IPV was 4X4 = 16 according to information available in 1974. The MEF score of OPV was not universally uniform – it varied between all developed countries on the one hand and several tropical developing countries on the other. The MEF score was 2.5X4 = 10 in developed countries and 2.5X3 = 7.5 in some developing countries (see Table 3.1). Developed countries did not depend on WHO for policy decisions on vaccine choice, but all developing countries had accepted the EPI design and its vaccine policy emanating from WHO. Therefore WHO had the moral responsibility to guide them – with science, evidence and ethics.

As WHO had already suspected in the 1960s – even before WHO assumed custodianship of Sabin viruses, there was a very serious problem on hand, of low efficacy of OPV – as we shall detail below. Despite the incomplete safety and suboptimal efficacy, inexplicably, WHO made the policy of exclusive use of OPV in EPI, without either giving some room for considering IPV, or even the gentlemanly kindness of a cautionary clause or warning – legitimately due, on safety and efficacy.

That ill-advised choice, closing the door against IPV, contained the seeds of the present serious problems, not one but two, facing the WHO and global polio eradication program – (1) of delay in eradicating wild virus polio globally, and (2) in creating too many cases of VAPP and "contact VAPP" that are sporadic and swept under the carpet by not registering them as polio, and outbreaks of polio due to "vaccine-derived polioviruses" (described below), not known in 1974 but an embarrassingly serious and common problem, currently.

Why did the two important problems of OPV, vaccine-failure in developing countries and serious adverse reaction to the vaccine universally, not ring ethics or human rights alarm bells about the exclusive use of OPV? This will remain as one of the worst examples of the paternalistic attitude of global experts who were mostly from USA and Europe, in the history of global public health. Minority voices of experts from developing countries or Scandinavian countries were not respected.

WHO knew of low OPV efficacy in tropical developing countries

Earlier, we had mentioned that Sabin himself had popularised OPV in many developing countries. The WHO was always a world-watcher of infectious diseases. By mid-1960s, the WHO had noticed a potential efficacy problem with OPV in two tropical countries, Singapore and Kenya.

The Professor and Head of the Department of Child Health in the Christian Medical College, Vellore, India, was John KG Webb from England. In 1967 he was flying back from England to India to return to Vellore from home leave. The flight had one stop in some city in Europe; the gentleman sitting next to John Webb introduced himself as Dr Chas Cockburn, Medical Officer for Viral Diseases, WHO, Geneva; he was travelling to Geneva. When he learned of John Webb's circumstances, he broached a technical subject.

WHO had information that in Singapore and in Kenya, OPV was not inducing poliovirus antibodies in children at the expected high frequency, compared to data from the USA and Europe. To Dr Cockburn, the reason was apparently obvious – OPV was getting damaged in the tropical heat and was losing potency. However, WHO wanted to confirm that was the case, and, asked John Webb if he knew someone in India to test that explanation. Yes, he knew and mentioned that a young paediatrician in South India, could test the hypothesis.

The above narrative is from the memory of conversation one of us, T Jacob John, had with Prof John Webb, soon after he reached back in Vellore. To continue in Dr John's words:

"Dr Cockburn invited me for a meeting in May 1968 in Helsinki, Finland. The meeting group consisted of Dr Cockburn (from Geneva), Dr Albert Sabin, Dr Joseph Melnick, Dr John Fox, Dr Montefiore, R Waldman (all from the USA), Dr Isamu

Tagaya (from Japan) Dr Oker Blom (from Finland) and myself (from India).

I provided new information – that an occasional child had developed polio in spite of taking three doses of OPV. Two such cases had already been documented with virological confirmation.

Question: *"Are you sure these children had polio?"*

Answer: *"Yes, indeed: stool samples of both children had poliovirus type 3".*

Question: "Was the polio wild virus polio or vaccine-associated paralytic polio?"

Answer: *"My lab does not have expertise or experience in differentiating between wild and vaccine viruses. But since polio onset was a few months after the last dose of OPV – clearly beyond the upper range of incubation period of VAPP, I felt that both children had wild virus polio due to vaccine-failure".*(Vaccine-failure is the term applied to the situation in which a 'fully vaccinated' child develops the disease. Three-dose vaccine-failure of OPV was unheard of, at that time.)

Question: *"Where did you get the vaccine from; how do you know if the vaccine was potent, or had not been inactivated in the tropical heat?"*

Answer: *"Dr John Webb had started giving OPV in CMC Vellore in 1964 because of the high prevalence of polio in children. It came from Wellcome or Pfizer Laboratories in England, flown directly to Madras, our nearest airport. As far as I have learned from the pharmacy, OPV was sent packed in some kind of special boxes with dry ice -- It was picked up in ice-containing boxes and brought to CMC where the pharmacy collected and kept the vaccine in good quality refrigerators. The Immunization Clinic that functioned twice every week was supplied with OPV in ice-containers and vaccine was always kept cold. Only small quantities were supplied – if stock ran out, more vaccine was brought from the pharmacy. One more piece of information -- after the first child with suspected vaccine-*

failure-polio was detected, immediately the vaccine in stock was sampled and tested in the virus lab and it had full potency of total virus content. I had not checked if types 1, 2 and 3 had the required potency but the total virus content was in the range of full potency. Since then vaccine potency was periodically measured and always found good".

A lot of discussions followed. If vaccine-failure occurred and the vaccine was fully potent, there must be some other reason than the loss of potency and vaccinated children remaining susceptible. The hypothesis that the vaccine had lost potency was already, almost, proved incorrect.

Humans are one species; polioviruses are universally the same. OPV contains infectious but attenuated polioviruses; in USA and Europe, 3 OPV doses immunise virtually 100% children. So, there was a riddle here, which needed to be solved.

Dr Melnick suggested that other enterovirus infections, very frequent in children, might have interfered with OPV 'take' (gut infection) and protective immune response. That was very plausible, but failure after three doses had never been seen anywhere else, particularly in rich countries. Enterovirus infections are common everywhere. Children in all parts of the world are likely to have some frequency of such infections when OPV is given – but three doses would have overcome any interference that might have occurred perhaps to any one dose. Anyway, that question needed to be tested in Vellore.

Dr Sabin suggested that maternal antibody in the infant's blood or in breast milk might be inhibiting vaccine virus take – as mothers would have high antibody levels from repeated wild virus infections. So he asked if we could defer vaccination to after one year when breastfeeding also will not be an interfering factor. My answer surprised him: infants were at risk of polio from about five months of age, and nearly half the children with polio had got polio before the first birthday. We discussed the old name of polio as 'infantile paralysis' – but half the cases in infancy was indeed a surprise. The upper age limit of polio in Vellore was five years.

The group's decision was to recommend to WHO to conduct a definitive study in Vellore using quality-assured vaccine and to measure the rate of antibody response. WHO would fund the entire study.

The study design and results were reported to the WHO annually from 1969 through 1972 and published as four papers – two in 1972 and 2 in 1975. The first, third and fourth were in American Journal of Epidemiology, [6,7,8] and the second in Indian Pediatrics.[4] The conclusions were: antibody response (seroconversion) rates were quite low compared to published results in temperate climate countries; loss of vaccine potency and interference from enteroviruses were ruled out as the reason.

The bottom line is that WHO staff/experts were well aware of the serious problem with the low frequency of antibody response of children in a few tropical countries – the Vellore study had confirmed sub-optimal antibody response to OPV. Moreover, its real-life consequence was demonstrated with clinical cases of vaccine-failure polio; in 1973, we had reported on six such cases seen in Vellore.[5]

These were not data that could simply be ignored, but they were ignored as evidenced by the 1974 EPI recommendation of only 3 doses of OPV in early infancy. The original recommendation was to give OPV at 8, 12 and 16 weeks, later amended to 6, 10 and 14 weeks.

Had the information on low OPV efficacy not been ignored, alternate tactics would have been sought and field-tested. In 1974 it was well known that in Scandinavian countries IPV was performing extremely well. Was the potential role of IPV considered and discarded or not at all considered? We do not know, and there seems to be no information on that. WHO's silence on IPV was loud enough for us to judge it as deliberate rejection.

Had WHO polio experts cared to compare OPV and IPV, the safety problem in all countries using OPV exclusively, and the efficacy problem in India and other tropical developing countries, would have been very obvious. We project a quantitative comparison, with MEF scores of 7.5 for OPV in tropical developing countries versus 16 for IPV wherever it was being used. The differential, although quantitatively not given MEF scores by others, was qualitatively widely known both to WHO experts and other polio experts globally.

The efficacy problem was widely known among Indian paediatricians and health administrators. As a sovereign country Government of India had the full freedom to decide its own policy – India also chose exclusively OPV for India EPI, launched in 1978. Apparently, the WHO policy heavily influenced government health administrators – who chose to ignore even Indian scientific data. Such was the influence of WHO on developing countries.

Was there any justification for OPV in EPI?

We believe, that in spite of the safety and efficacy problems of OPV, and its low MEF score, there was some justification for the choice of OPV in EPI, but only for a short period and with a caveat.

We had alluded to non-MEF qualities of vaccines such as low cost, ease of administration and benefit-risk assessment. EPI was truly a great program created by WHO, to popularise vaccines against six serious diseases among children – often called killer diseases – childhood tuberculosis, diphtheria, pertussis (whooping cough), tetanus (both neonatal and beyond infancy), polio and measles.

All the other vaccines in EPI schedule, namely BCG, DPT and measles vaccine were injected. This oral vaccine, OPV, saved (or avoided) one additional injection, as the timing of the schedule, three doses, coincided with that of 3 injections of DPT. If IPV was to be used, one additional injection, three times, would be needed. That meant two injections at one clinic visit. Mothers might not have liked it. At that time, no combined DPT-plus-IPV had been made. A decade later, such combination vaccine became available, but neither WHO nor Government of India seized the opportunity to include it in EPI. When the combination vaccine of DPT-IPV (quadrivalent vaccine) became available, it could and should have been factored into EPI, but it was not.

In the 1980s, based on the low MEF score of OPV, and particularly due to ethical impropriety, a sunset plan for OPV with increasing use of IPV would have been the wise and correct course for WHO and India as well, and for other developing countries that were guided by WHO policies, as was recommended in a journal editorial in 1981.[9]

In 1984, a quadrivalent vaccine of DPT-IPV was available in Europe and also successfully manufactured in India, but its production was stopped by the government.[10] The exclusion of IPV by policy was against the best interests of, not only developing countries, but also WHO itself as history has taught us. Currently, a six-component (hexavalent) vaccine is available -- containing DPT, IPV, Hepatitis B vaccine and *H influenzae* b vaccine.

In addition to low cost and ease of giving, another reason justifying the exclusive use of OPV for a limited period was the potential of the favourable benefit-risk equation at that point of time. That limited period of time should have been used to rapidly reduce the burden of polio in countries adopting EPI, and also for planning to introduce IPV in all developing countries.

The burden of polio at that time was disturbingly high, although not measured in most low-income countries. In the Vellore CMC paediatric clinic, polio was a very common disease. While the Government of India had not begun promoting polio immunization, the head of paediatrics, Dr JKG Webb, had taken his own initiative to import OPV and inoculate children who came to the clinic. This he started in 1964. From 1966 when one of us was working in CMC Vellore, we were admitting about one polio case per week – only children in distress were admitted -- children with just one limb paralysed and not in distress were cared for at home with instructions from the clinic.

Our orthopaedic colleagues were busy operating on children with deformities due to polio. They had assessed that some 30% of all orthopaedic work was for polio corrective surgery. Polio was a big problem.

In the 1970s and 1980s, we had documented the very high *'annual incidence'* (number of new cases per unit population per year) of polio. In both urban and rural communities, the incidence was about 20-25 per 100,000 people per year.[11] We extrapolated and projected 200,000 cases per year in India, during those years. In one epidemic year, the incidence in Delhi was 40 per 100,000 per year – for 400,000 cases in India in one year.[12] The average daily polio burden was about 500 in most years and about 1000 in some years.

Another measure we used was polio lameness survey among school children – 6-8 among 1000 school children in grades 1 to 5 had lameness due to polio.[13,14]

Against this background, OPV, due to its low cost and ease of administration, was potentially an immediate solution to the problem.[9] As far as India was concerned, already there was an indigenous OPV manufacturing facility in Coonoor, Tamil Nadu, India, established with help and guidance from Sabin himself.

Sadly, all these did not happen. The WHO EPI did not advise the rapid control of polio, or any other disease targeted for prevention under EPI (except for neonatal tetanus).

For disease control, disease surveillance is essential. For neonatal tetanus, there was a simple method – counting death of neonates within 28 days of birth with certain clinical criteria. Such cases were deemed to be neonatal tetanus. For all other diseases, surveillance had to be community-based and nested within primary healthcare. EPI did not have a design of concentric expansion to grow into universal primary healthcare.

India considered OPV similar to other injected vaccines and introduced it with slow build-up. The real advantage of oral feeding was to de-link it from other injected vaccines and to go on a mass scale – as the problem was 500-1000 cases of polio per day. EPI did not include a disease burden monitoring mechanism – therefore, it remained a vaccine-delivery platform rather than a disease-control program.[15] For disease control, disease surveillance would have been essential. That was not planned in EPI. In the absence of polio surveillance not only was polio not targeted for control, but in addition it was easy to sweep VAPP cases under the carpet.

India had a method of monitoring disease burden trends based on 'sentinel' institutions. The sentinel institutions were a number of selected large government hospitals with good laboratory infrastructure. They collected and passed on data on a few diseases, selected by the government. The objective was to follow disease burden trends over time. It had been assumed that they collectively represented roughly 10% of the national disease burdens.

According to the reports of sentinel hospitals, polio burden actually increased during the years immediately after launching EPI and did not decline to pre-EPI level for more than a decade from the year we started India EPI.[16] Therefore our justification for exclusive OPV policy by WHO as applied at least to India did not become valid—neither WHO nor the Government of India appeared keen to control polio expeditiously.

Moreover, in a bizarre and self-defeating manner, the one and only OPV manufacturing facility in India was ordered closed in 1974. India had never again succeeded in indigenously manufacturing OPV, in spite of many and repeated attempts in several institutions.

Since the justification for OPV – the potential of rapid control of polio using OPV -- was not fulfilled, the continued policy of the exclusive use of OPV in EPI was no longer justifiable on account of poor efficacy and problems of safety reflected in the very low MEF score.

MEF scores in 1988 as polio eradication was launched

The spirit of the 1988 resolution for the global eradication of polio was to nest the program within EPI. Unfortunately, EPI had the policy of using OPV and only OPV. Thus the global polio eradication program inherited the flawed immunization policy of EPI, from which it has not yet fully recovered.

By 1988 the fact that the efficacy problem was widespread in many more tropical developing countries was well known, and a comprehensive review of the global picture was published in 1991.[15] The efficacy problem in many developing countries was proved beyond question. The efficacy score of 3 was still appropriate and realistic, justified, in those countries, in 1988. But that was not the last word on efficacy score of OPV or of its MEF score.

Regarding safety: VAPP in the vaccinated and "contact VAPP" were found to be occurring in all countries using OPV, by the WHO study in Europe.[3,18] A new safety problem was had been recognised post-1974. Immuno-deficient children (and adults), were prone to prolonged intestinal carriage of vaccine viruses (but not wild polioviruses) and were also highly susceptible to developing VAPP.[19]

Today we know that such viruses in immune-deficient persons are 'vaccine-derived polioviruses' with regained neurovirulence. Such polioviruses are called 'immunodeficiency-associated VDPV' or iVDPV. This is a very strange phenomenon. Chronic infection with wild polioviruses does not occur in immune-deficient persons, but it does with vaccine viruses. That gave us a message that the immune system was able to clearly discriminate between wild and vaccine polioviruses.

There is another piece of relevant information. Many reports were showing that the viruses shed by normal children after they were given OPV, were already more neurovirulent than vaccine viruses in the vials. That itself was a clear danger signal. If vaccinated children were shedding more neurovirulent viruses and if they infected other children, the consequences would be sinister. By the year 2000 we knew that such viruses are capable of seeding the emergence of virulent vaccine-derived polioviruses (VDPVs). Such VDPVs may circulate in the community, having regained transmission efficiency that was minimised through attenuation. Circulating VDPVs (cVDPVs) are capable of causing polio outbreaks, as we describe below.

Because of these four additional safety problems – (1) chronic infection in immune-deficient persons, (2) unacceptable frequency of VAPP in immune-deficient children and adults, and (3) increasing neuro-virulence in laterally transmitted vaccine viruses, and (4) the emergence of cVDPVs -- the safety score of 2.5 was no longer justified – that score was over-estimated. It should have been lower – we reduce it to 2 (see Table 4.1).

In summary, the global polio eradication program faced the choice between IPV with MEF score of 16 and OPV with MEF score of 2X3 = 6 in many tropical developing countries. Yet, the policy of the program was the exclusive use of OPV – the most likely reasons were some kind of psychological 'path-fixation'; bias in favour of OPV with proprietary ownership held by WHO; inexplicable hubris of faith in OPV; the irrational expectation that the problems of OPV may self-correct if time was given; the erroneous belief that inducing intestinal mucosal immunity was essential for interrupting the transmission of wild polioviruses; or something we have not figured out.

For OPV to induce intestinal mucosal immunity, it ought to have high efficacy score. OPV did not have a high score. How could a vaccine that does not immunise a majority of children with 3-4 doses be expected to induce intestinal immunity in them?

On the other hand, IPV had high efficacy score. Moreover, retardation of wild virus transmission locally with IPV had been demonstrated in the USA. Interruption of wild virus transmission, nation-wide, had been shown in Finland, Sweden, Norway and Iceland. We are not aware of any evaluation conducted by the eradication program to support the belief that OPV was essential and IPV was incapable of interrupting wild virus transmission. Was not the choice of the vaccine in the strategy of eradication made on faith and not evidence?

Safety and efficacy scores of OPV and IPV in the 21st century

Since 1988, yet another safety problem of OPV had occurred, ignored first, and surfaced again in 2000. The signals of that safety problem were present from the early times but missed by most experts. What was 'community-acquired VAPP'? VAPP and "contact VAPP" were known and explained as a consequence of regaining of virulence – we have an alternate explanation that will be presented later. 'Community-acquired VAPP', known from 1964, was a signal that vaccine virus could laterally spread and very occasionally circulate in the community so that some unsuspecting child gets infected and be paralysed. The semantic problem of calling the transmitted virus as vaccine virus was pointed out earlier.

So, there was potential for vaccine-virus spreading, circulating and turning wild-like, causing outbreaks of polio. One such outbreak was detected in Egypt – lasting a decade, from 1983 to 1993.[20] The second was in 2000, in the Dominican Republic and adjoining Haiti.[21] This time the semantic problem was faced squarely, and the virus was named vaccine-derived, qualified as "circulating vaccine-derived poliovirus" (cVDPV).[21]

Cases of 'community-acquired VAPP' actually had signalled that Sabin viruses could circulate silently until polio paralysis was manifest in someone. That was exemplified in one major episode, Egypt. For the sake of argument that episode could have been dismissed as just a one-off event -- an exception to the rule. The second episode, the Dominican Republic and Haiti polio outbreak confirmed that it was the rule and not the exception. One swallow may not signal summer but if even two do not convince, there is a serious problem.

Had there not been an eradication program, these episodes could be taken only as a trigger to monitor the global scene to detect such episodes in countries using OPV. As the eradication program was in full swing but had failed the time target in 2000, these two episodes were an alarm bell, loud and clear, that more episodes were to be expected. Clearly, OPV was not compatible with global polio eradication. With this additional safety problem, the program had an obligation to review the situation in 2000-2001 and plan for the introduction of IPV in developing countries at the earliest. The safety score of OPV was to be further reduced from 2 to 1.5.

So MEF score of OPV was now $1.5 \times 3 = 4.5$ in 2001, as against that of IPV at 16. Polio experts of the eradication program remained unmoved. It was scientifically, morally and philosophically no longer justified to have insisted on the exclusive use of OPV for polio eradication since the Haiti-Dominican Republic episode of the emergence of cVDPV polio outbreak was observed, investigated, understood.

When the target year of 2000 came and passed by, OPV, one of the two causes of polio, both sporadic and outbreak, had to be stopped and all fight should have been exclusively against natural (wild) polioviruses. Eradication tactics should have been designed WPV-centric and not OPV-centric.

Table 3.1: *Comparison of estimated Minimum Essential Function (MEF) Scores of OPV and IPV in developed and developing countries in the years 1974 (when EPI was launched), 1988 (when polio eradication program was launched) and 2001 (after the original target for polio eradication was missed in 2000)*

	Year	OPV			IPV		
		Safety	Efficacy	Product	Safety	Efficacy	Product
		a	b	axb	c	d	cxd
Maximum score of MEF		4	4	16	4	4	16
Developed countries	1974	2.5*	4	10	4	4	16
	1988	2$	4	8	4	4	16
	2001	1.5^	4	6	4	4	16
Developing countries	1974	2.5*	3+	7.5	4	4	16
	1988	2$	3+	6	4	4	16
	2001	1.5^	3+	4.5	4	4	16

* *Low score due to adverse events, namely VAPP in the vaccinated and in contacts*
+ *Low score due to low antibody responses and vaccine failure polio cases*
$ *Very low score due to emergence of VDPVs*

^ *Lowest score due to outbreaks of Community acquired VAPP in Egypt (1983 to 1993) and Haiti-Dominican Republic (2000), in other words, cVDPV.*

Contact and Community-acquired VAPP are not vaccine adverse reactions

Vaccine adverse reactions are, by definition, in vaccinated children. The problems of sporadic VAPP among close contacts of vaccinated children ("contact VAPP"), "community-acquired VAPP" and polio outbreaks in the community due to vaccine-derived viruses, are *sensu stricto,* not 'vaccine adverse reactions' since they occur not in the vaccinated, but in unvaccinated individuals.

They are the most problematic, worrisome and sinister consequence of the exclusive and widespread use of OPV. Public health ethics do not allow collateral damage to uninvolved parties, when a safe alternative weapon was always available for the war. More detailed assessment of ethical problems of the continued use of OPV will be discussed in a chapter dedicated to ethical issues.

OPV unsafe at any dose

The clinical definition of 'VAPP in the vaccinated' is paralytic polio developing within 4 to 30 days after OPV feeding by mouth.

The incubation period of wild virus polio is also 4-30 days. In other words, the incubation periods of VAPP in the vaccinated and of wild virus polio are identical. Paralytic disease is rare with vaccine virus infection, but more common with wild virus infection. That means, the main difference between VAPP and wild virus polio is the 'case-to-infection' ratio, higher for wild virus and lower for vaccine virus. The clinical disease is identical whether caused by wild virus or vaccine virus and incubation period, an integral element of clinical disease, is also identical. If one in 1000 wild-virus infected children develops polio, and one in 1,000,000 vaccine virus-infected children develops polio, without a shift in the range of incubation period, we may make the following conclusions.

Wild polioviruses are already naturally 'attenuated,' so to say, causing paralysis quite infrequently. Vaccine polioviruses are 'further attenuated' causing paralysis even more infrequently, or shall we say very rarely? Using OPV, when we prevent 1000 cases of wild-virus polio, inevitably we will cause one case of VAPP in the vaccinated. Without going into details, this frequency of thousand wild-virus polio prevented for the price of one VAPP is roughly correct in many countries.

The second conclusion is about the neurovirulence of wild versus vaccine viruses. When a child gets infected with the wild virus, we know that it is already neurovirulent, and can cause polio paralysis within five days in some children and within 31 days in all others. For fully neurovirulent viruses, the range of 4-30 days is its natural range. When VAPP also has the same range of incubation period as 4 to 30 days, it is obvious that the vaccine from the vial already contained viruses that could cause paralysis – in other words, already neurovirulent.

The incubation period of 4 days, even one or two weeks, is too short for mutations to occur, and then invade the body tissues, including the spinal cord, and then cause paralysis. If the very first viruses that invaded the body tissues were totally non-neurovirulent, they would be the ones that kick-start immune responses. Immune responses occur within a few days, and thereafter even if neurovirulent mutated viruses were present in the intestine of the child, they would not be able to cause paralysis. What we surmise is that the vaccine drops in the vial itself must have had neurovirulent mutants in order for a child to get paralysed with a short incubation period. Could the vaccine in the vial have neurovirulent viruses?

The general teaching is that vaccine polioviruses are genetically unstable, and mutations tend to occur as they multiply in the child. Consequently, the mutated viruses, those that acquired neurovirulence while multiplying in the child, were the cause of polio, but not the original viruses from the vaccine vial. This seems to exonerate the vaccine in the vial from the guilt of causing paralysis, but it was the virus that grew in the child's body that was to be blamed. Wrong.

Mutations do occur in the vaccinated child but these mutated vaccine viruses, rather than affecting the same, now immune child, get shed though the child's faeces into the environment. Such faecal shedding of mutated virus can be diagnosed by faecal sampling and testing, but epidemiologically they have reached a dead-end, as faecal-oral spread is most unlikely for polioviruses, as we explain in Chapter 6.

That is a fact: every dose of OPV from the vial, already contains, a very small number of neurovirulent viruses. [22,23] Thus, it is the very low proportion of neurovirulent viruses in the vaccine that causes polio at very low frequency in the vaccinated children.

Unless a neurovirulent virus entered the body tissue first, polio paralysis is unlikely to occur. If non-virulent (attenuated) virus enters first, it will spread widely within the body and disease will not ensue. In a short time, immune responses will manifest within the body, and thereafter the virulent virus in the vaccine cannot cause disease. This is a theoretical explanation. If virulent viruses are distributed in the vial such that only one in a thousand is neurovirulent, then the probability of a neurovirulent virus entering the body tissue first is once in 1000 vaccine feedings. Each dose of OPV contains 1,000,000 live type 1 viruses and 600,000 type 3 viruses. Arithmetic calculation of one in 1000 chance of neurovirulent virus infecting vaccinated children should explain polio due to type 3 virus in one in 1000X600 =1/600,000 vaccinated children. For type 1, the probability of one VAPP in the vaccinated among 1,000X1000 = 1/1,000,000 vaccinated children. Sabin type 2 virus has the least risk for VAPP, but the most risk for "contact-VAPP". In the USA one in 750,000 children given OPV was the frequency of VAPP caused by types 1 or 3.

If the virus that multiplies in the vaccinated child was neurovirulent, then the probability of throat shedding will be higher, leading to transmission to contact children, explaining "contact-VAPP". Since "contact VAPP" is the fore-runner of polio outbreak due to cVDPV, type 2 Sabin virus is by far the commonest cause of cVDPV polio outbreak. Just as motor cars are very safe, but when unsafe, they can be unsafe at any speed, OPV is very safe, but when unsafe it can be unsafe at any dose.

Summation

Choices indeed are the hinges of destiny. Small choices by big organisations can have big consequences. In health-care, a wrong choice is called medical negligence. It adversely affects one person. When applying public health interventions, the choice may not appear to be of crucial significance, as between OPV and IPV, two vaccines used in different countries, but experts who make the choice on a global level have the moral responsibility to be objective, serious-minded without any trace of bias, strictly following scientific and ethical principles to the last detail. Otherwise 'public health negligence' with consequences on many may ensue. Polio eradication was destined to succeed by 2000 if the right choices were made at right times. Wrong choices, one leading to another – exclusive use of OPV, leading to the escape of the eradication program out of the EPI platform; escaping from the strict domain of the cognitive into the belief-domain; ignoring the sinister consequences of the very first wrong choice; all have conspired together to deny destiny's due success intended for polio eradication by the year 2000.

§§§

Section Two

The two polio vaccines were an unusual global asset. Unfortunately, good opportunities appeared to have been missed in utilising this asset in the best interests of humanity.

The two vaccines had somewhat opposite qualities, the deficiencies of the one with flaws could elegantly be covered by the other, in order to exploit the advantages of both for the benefit of children in all developing countries.

Instead, they, not all but the ones in decision-making role for the world of developing countries, took the very narrow view that the contrasting qualities must spell contradictory attributes, for which reason one had to be rejected and the other accepted. Other polio experts who understood the error, in European nations that had wisely chosen the one vaccine with full marks for safety and efficacy, remained a silent minority, excluded from policy-making echelons of global polio eradication.

4. JONAS SALK AND THE INACTIVATED POLIOVIRUS VACCINE

Edward R Murrow: *Who owns the patent of this vaccine?*

Jonas Salk: *Well, the people, I would say. There is no patent. Could you patent the Sun?*

CBC Television Interview, on See It Now; 12 April 1955

Why was the one vaccine, IPV, which could predictably prevent and control polio in rich as well as low-income countries, hence eradicate polio globally, as shown by proof of principle, pilot projects and scientific reasoning, not included in the armamentarium of this ill-fated war on polio? The reason can only be figured out by recapitulating the story behind the vaccine, the scientist who created it and how both were perceived by peers.

The reason was not scientific but spurious, hence outside the realm of reasoning and logic. It can be understood when we learn the stories behind both IPV and OPV, and Jonas Salk and Albert Sabin.

The development, demonstration of efficacy and safety and licensing and distribution of IPV was truly a landmark event in the global history of public health, in the country known as the Mecca of public health, the USA. That event marked science's potential victory in the war against polio – akin to another landmark two centuries earlier, the gathering of scientific proof that 'vaccinia' inoculation (smallpox vaccination) predictably prevented smallpox.

The polio landmark event was in 1954-55 -- a mammoth vaccine trial starting in 1954 and culminating in the formal announcement, in a theatrical public meeting, on 12 April 1955, that it was completely safe and highly effective in protecting children from polio. The same day it was licensed in the USA. Vaccine manufacturers had been pre-prepared to roll out the vaccine at the shortest notice. Polio began rapidly declining in numbers.

The entry of OPV in the USA while IPV was still in use

Then in 1961, the live attenuated oral polio vaccine was licensed in the USA 'believing' (without ascertaining) that it was completely safe and highly effective.

The majority of medical and public health professionals were enamoured by OPV, blurring their cold objectivity. During the next seven years, medical and paediatric professional associations, public health leaders and policymakers increasingly recommended its use. In 1964 the national policy began shifting from IPV to OPV, as the trivalent OPV became available. In 1968 the national policy insisted on the exclusive use of OPV. Manufacturing of IPV was abandoned in the USA. All these, due to the imagined or believed superiority of OPV over IPV.

During this interval, trivalent OPV's efficacy was confirmed to be virtually 100%, whereas its safety was clearly recognised not to be so. Every year on an average, some ten children developed polio caused by vaccine viruses in OPV. However, the policy did not shift back to IPV. That by itself was strange, and it signalled an attitudinal flaw.

Countries that looked up to the USA for guidance in public health got the message that something was not right with IPV, but OPV was the vaccine of choice against polio. The damage was already done.

Schismatic policies on IPV and OPV in USA

The first generation IPV that was tested in the mammoth vaccine evaluation of 1954 had clearly shown that its efficacy after three doses was high, but not near 100%. The vaccine trial also clearly showed that the antigen content of IPV made by different companies varied and that protective efficacy was proportional to, hence determined by, the vaccine potency. That stands to reason. The logical, scientific, next step, should have been aimed at improving the potency, standardising potency across manufacturers, and, defining the best schedule of vaccine doses.

But instead, the USA rejected IPV, and its manufacture stopped in the US. The work avoided by the US was done by the Dutch in the 1980s, and since then we have the perfect vaccine against polio – the enhanced potency IPV, just two doses of which gives virtually 100% immunity. Perfect, on the basis of complete safety and exquisite efficacy.

The rejection of IPV and the acceptance of OPV in the USA were not based on epidemiology or economics and were clearly contrary to ethics – but what was the basis of the choice? To the best of our assessment, from reading the history of the policy shift in the USA, that choice of the vaccine was based on the choice between Salk and Sabin as the real 'knight in white armour' who defeated polio. That was unnecessary and incredible, particularly coming from the country known as the Mecca of public health. Polio scientists and public health leaders deified Sabin but demonised Salk – and the vaccine called Salk vaccine had to be rejected. They couldn't reject Salk but accept Salk vaccine – they could have, but we humans are slaves to our prejudices and tendencies to invent false justifications of wrong decisions already made.

There was another unseen problem – should non-medical people representing the public decide or should scientists and public health leaders decide? Scientists are jealous guardians of the rituals, rules and processes of scientific endeavours. Salk vaccine belonged to the public; Sabin vaccine belonged to science (read scientists).

That the merits and disadvantages of the two vaccines remained controversial in the US is widely recognised – but as it was in the country of origin of both vaccines, the lesson for the rest of the world, the WHO included, was, that IPV ought to be rejected and OPV embraced. Bizarre – who suffered the consequence of the choice by way of vaccine-caused polio? Well, obviously the public, the owners of IPV; did they deserve to be punished?

There was yet another issue: national public health leaders who decided on licensing of OPV without ascertaining its safety were the very officials who had to take a call -- on its continued use after detecting its safety problem, or, its withdrawal, or at least suspension pending investigation. The very first year, there were 24 paralysed children due to OPV. We referred to the human tendency for justification, even if contrived, to prove wrong decision as right.

Hans Christian Anderson's Emperor, when he found out that he was foolish enough to have believed he had splendid clothes on, did not crouch or run back to the palace. Instead, he held his head even higher, and marched on, as if he had been correct all along.

Most officials, when confronted with an error of judgment, would tend to vehemently defend the earlier decision. For years, apparently, the polio eradication program has a similar dilemma, having declared from the start an OPV-only policy for eradication.

Hatred of Salk, anger at the public for the adulation of Salk – these two led to prejudice and bias in the minds of those in influential positions of power, the short term result of which was 'the baby thrown with the bathwater'. Why did the US not use both vaccines? In 1964 paediatricians in the US knew that even a single dose of IPV protected against vaccine-virus polio caused by OPV. It was a common practice to give one dose of Salk vaccine before giving OPV.

The long term result of the US policy of exclusive use of OPV and the exclusion of IPV from the national immunization schedule is that global polio eradication became OPV-centric. Therefore the safety problems of OPV had to be ignored. Actually, denied rather than ignored.

We consider that a polio eradicated world will be one that has no polio, caused by polioviruses, wild or vaccine, hence one that uses IPV exclusively and OPV is completely excluded from use. The earlier that is accepted by everyone, the better it is for the world.

WHO championed OPV from the beginning

In 1974, when the WHO launched the Expanded Program on Immunization, OPV was included and IPV excluded. No choice was given to countries. In 1988 when WHO spearheaded global polio eradication, again the policy was to use OPV exclusively. The exclusion of IPV from the armamentarium of polio eradication had, as we argue in this book, a lot to do with the subsequent delays and problems faced by the global polio eradication program.

Therefore the background and reasons for not including IPV in EPI and polio eradication program are extremely important for our understanding of the history of the problems and delays of polio eradication.

When the USA and WHO discredited IPV and chose OPV for exclusive use, public health leaders in many other countries read the message that IPV was not a good vaccine.

India for example accepted OPV in its EPI established in 1978 and refrained from licensing IPV until after the wind began blowing in its favour; India licensed IPV only in 2006, allowing its use in private sector pediatric practice, not for children depending on government sector healthcare and EPI.

Eventually, when polio eradication program leaders decided to withdraw Sabin virus type 2 from OPV, in 2016, they knew that it was a dangerous step, as the risk of development and spread of circulating vaccine-derived poliovirus type 2 (cVDPV-2) seeding new outbreaks of polio had been proved real. The only safe way forward was to give IPV first and then withdraw type 2; but how many doses?

The old USA experience was one dose of IPV to prevent VAPP. But there was a problem; due to the presence of maternal antibodies in young infants, IPV was more effective at or after 14 weeks of age, not earlier. Immunization program required a dose of OPV soon after birth and one dose each at 6, 10 and 14 weeks. So one dose of IPV was prescribed at 14 weeks, in order to mitigate the risk of emergence/spread of cVDPV-2. There was no precedent or scientific evidence that such a schedule would mitigate the risk of cVDPV – the later unfolding of events proved that the risk was not eliminated. However, one dose at 14 weeks, along with the third OPV dose, was the prescription.

Everyone knew it as an incomplete IPV schedule being used – enough to prime the immune system but not to provide near-100 per cent protection for the long term. Why such 'tight rope walking'? Was there not the probability that polio would be eradicated with full immunizing schedule of IPV? Was there a hidden agenda that such an eventuality ought to be avoided? Was there a stubborn determination that polio eradication must be achieved and seen to be achieved with OPV, only OPV, and not IPV?

The prescription meant all countries in the world that had not yet licensed IPV had to do so hurriedly. All countries complied. The conclusion is inevitable: countries without strong scientific background or expertise fully depended on WHO guidance and recommendations. Success or failure can be laid at one doorstep – that of WHO.

We propose that the failure to achieve polio eradication either on time (the year 2000), or within a reasonable time (say, latest by the year 2005) was the consequence of not using IPV in an appropriate and timely manner. When the USA shifted policy, why was the global polio eradication program not moved to reason and reality, and follow suit? Does that not mean that USA experts were not the major influencers of the program's policy?

As an introduction to the story of the beginnings of IPV, we will first present the OPV-IPV conundrum and the problems thereof. We will also present some of the problems of OPV that WHO experts knew about, but chose to ignore (read deny), even before launching EPI.

Everything under the sun has a reason. Our purpose is only to search for the reason, not to find fault for the sake of fault-finding. We are just interested in facts and their interpretation, and we are searching for answers to questions. We need that insight in order to suggest course-correction to expedite and ensure global polio eradication.

Along with such preliminaries, we will present the story of Jonas Salk and IPV, alluding to the origins and reasons of the OPV-IPV controversy conundrum. That story is one of its kind in all history of public health and vaccinology. The aversion to IPV on the part of the policymakers and public health experts in the USA was vicariously transferred from an intense dislike of the man after whom the vaccine was named – Salk. Much has been written about all this, but we will present it again in our own viewpoint and words.

Salk, a much misunderstood and maligned man

The technical expertise and design of the inactivated poliovirus vaccine were Salk's, but the maneuvering of the raw laboratory product into a vaccine that went for the world's largest vaccine trial for safety and efficacy, was neither Salk's doing nor under Salk's leadership – it was done by a man, lawyer by profession, polio-fighter with passion and obsession, Basil O'Conner. It was not meant as, but it turned out to be, an affront on established polio scientists.

Or, perhaps O'Connor knew very well that many scientists behaved as if science was a religion with its dogmas and rituals – but he was aiming for the greater goal of science – to save children from polio paralysis as early as possible. Delay meant more children paralysed. That was against the soul of science; that was against humanity.

In 2020 we stare at the COVID-19 pandemic and marvel at the speed with which vaccine candidates were developed and field-tested. How much evidence for safety and efficacy would suffice for vaccine rollout? Should the strict adherence to norms made for non-pandemic peace time be insisted upon, or are global public health leaders trust-worthy enough to modify norms for pandemic war-time and expedite vaccine rollout? For the individuals at high risk of severe disease and threat of death, protection delayed may turn out to be protection denied, resulting in death.

How O'Connor faced a similar situation is educative. The promoter of polio vaccine was a public trust, with absolutely no commercial profit motive. Financial investment was not by any vaccine company. Companies were invited to manufacture the vaccine on condition that all production over two years was paid for (advance purchase agreement in current parlance), with no financial risk to the companies. O'Conner understood that for many children approaching the next season of polio outbreak in the US, protection delayed would mean protection denied. It is when the 'good' is not trustworthy that we insist on 'perfection'.

O'Connor had done an immense amount of work to defeat polio that had become a scourge as it struck healthy children without any warning. He had been associated with Franklin D Roosevelt as a law partner. Roosevelt had been paralysed below the waist by polio. Yet he went on to become US President a record four times. After years of struggle (in vain) to help Roosevelt recover, their efforts changed direction to fight polio as a crippling disease in the country. *"On 23 September, 1937 at O'Connor's urging, Roosevelt announced the formation of the National Foundation for Infantile Paralysis, to be incorporated the following January"* [1]O'Connor was appointed as the President of the Foundation.

O'Connor was all hell-bent on finding a solution to polio. He began dreaming of, and hoping for, a vaccine to prevent polio. He raised enormous funds and generously provided them to many polio scientists for research on polio, with the goal of developing a vaccine. As soon as Salk provided the proof of principle of a vaccine and a product that was safe and immunogenic in humans, O'Connor saw its potential, urgency and timeliness. He grabbed the opportunity. No time 'wasted'. He virtually snatched the vaccine-candidate from Salk and ran with it to the finish line of licensing.

O'Connor had broken many rituals of science and in the process upset many established polio scientists. The large scale vaccine trial was conducted by Thomas Francis Jr. a widely respected epidemiologist, but not one among established polio scientists. His fame came from the Influenza vaccine. He had also worked on polio but not in-depth. But he did a superb job in the polio vaccine trial, but he also broke important rituals of science by going public with the results of the vaccine trial. Did they, O'Connor and Francis do these knowingly or unknowingly? If their actions were calculated and deliberate, they did what they did, most probably – or rather obviously, knowingly.

Francis himself was a great scientist – for him to have broken the rituals of first publishing the study results, and then going public, must have been after considerable soul-searching. Quite possibly, O'Connor would have convinced him of the reason: to expedite the licensing of the vaccine. Had the vaccine been dud, the publication would have been the next step. In the forenoon of 12 August 1955, the results were announced in a public meeting to which global media had been invited. The same afternoon the vaccine was licensed in the US. Was not quick licensing the intended result of the public announcement of the trial result?

Salk also broke rituals of science by allowing others to further the progress of the vaccine he developed. Conventionally the creator of the vaccine is expected to develop a candidate vaccine to a testable product and to conduct a vaccine trial by himself. Then he should publish the results in a peer-reviewed journal. All blame for all such unconventional steps was directed at Jonas Salk, suspecting that he was the mastermind behind what O'Connor was doing. O'Connor was the real mastermind behind Salk.

Most probably, they all knew that O'Connor was the mastermind, but he was not a card-holding member of the science-religion. Thomas Francis was an established and respected scientist – famous for his work on influenza in the time of the Second World War. No one dared to raise a finger at him regarding the manner in which the trial result was announced as a media event. Salk was a light-weight and easy target, like a fly on the same side of the glass for the jumping spider. He had 'betrayed' science by flouting rules and rituals of scientists. So, he came to be depicted by peer scientists as someone that he was not; demonised, in essence. Conquering polio at the earliest was not important to them. Then what was science for?

It was obvious that the rituals of scientists were more important to them than saving children from paralysis – O'Connor had the exact opposite view. Strange, that no important scientist (except Francis) seemed to appreciate the need for super-fast speed for getting the vaccine out to the public. That speed was achieved by Basil O'Connor, Thomas Francis and Jonas Salk by breaking rituals and going straight to the prevention of polio.

Were rituals made for science and scientists or science and scientists made for rituals? Didn't scientists have compassion? The result of short-cutting of rituals was to save hundreds of children from polio paralysis the very earliest. Polio season – May to November -- was just about to begin in the US. We are talking about events in April. What was truly more important to scientists, prevention of polio or strict adherence to rituals?

The consequence of the success of the vaccine was that Salk became a public hero and was adulated by the public. It was then easy to accuse him of wanting public adulation instead of acceptance by peer scientists.

Salk was relatively a newcomer to polio research – just five years earlier, in 1949, he was beginning to have some experience with polioviruses. Imagine that: just five years from scratch to vaccine – a world record. That could not have been achieved by the slow process of science advancing step by step. What was the driving force of Salk and O'Connor? Could it have been the monumental mission in mind – to create a vaccine against polio in the shortest time?

There were established polio researchers of standing over several decades. They were also working on developing a vaccine against polio for quite a number of years.

Albert Sabin was one of them. You could imagine the dismay and disappointment of the established polio scientists when they were overtaken by a lightweight novice. They were finding fault with everything connected with Salk and his vaccine.

But Salk was no novice – he was a scientist with a revolutionary concept of vaccinology. He probably was too naive to understand the reasons and magnitude of the ill feelings of virtually all leading polio scientists of the day. Or perhaps he understood, but even one child protected from polio was worth its heavy price. The fact that Salk quit his laboratory pursuits immediately after getting the vaccine licensed was his deliberate decision. That alone is sufficient for us to guess, understand and judge his thinking. He stood no chance of acceptance among the established polio scientists, and he must have understood, accepted. In the religion of science Salk was the saint of polio prevention, many others sinners.

1980 Boston Marathon, women's race: Rosie Ruiz reached the finish line ahead of everyone else. Marathon officials later discovered that she had not started at the starting line, but joined the runners about 2 kilometres before the finish line. Her victory was false; she was disqualified; Jacqueline Gareau was declared the winner. The 'ignominy' of Salk was somewhat like that of Rosa Ruiz, except that Salk's was not in a sports race with others. Salk had done everything right. Salk's victory was legitimate. Polio was conquered. But Salk had not been a 'recognized' contestant in the race for a vaccine. In fact, O'Conner and Francis ran the race on behalf of the vaccine – others felt that they did that on behalf of Salk. Scientists were confused, turned uncharitable, and abandoned some of their own rules of honesty and objectivity, the need for evidence -- and the soul of science.

The race was over and polio conquered. Salk retired from science as a celebrity, a popular idol, described the second greatest human in the twentieth century after Albert Einstein – he had to retire because he was *ipso facto* excommunicated by the high priests of polio science and public health.

Faith in live vaccine over evidence of killed virus

For the established polio scientists the race was not over yet – as they all wanted a live virus vaccine – they had set their own finishing line. Among a few top scientists working on a live vaccine, Sabin succeeded to develop the best vaccine virus strains a few years after Salk vaccine's licensure, working double-time as Salk's vaccine was already in use and rapidly reducing the burden of polio.

Scientists and public health leaders in the USA declared Sabin the winner of the race as he had developed the vaccine of their faith. As soon as Sabin's vaccine became available, after some early hiccups, they formally accepted it in the country without a vaccine trial or even careful assessment of its safety. Even when found not completely safe, they stuck to their guns.

Science was played down, ethics abandoned. These set of events changed the direction of the future course of polio prevention, control, elimination, eradication. Not for better, but for worse – but that is a matter of opinion, our opinion.

Facts can be stranger than fiction. Salk had wanted (based on science and logic) a killed virus vaccine against a virus disease, particularly for assured safety, while most scientists wanted (based on belief) that only a live virus vaccine should be used against polio. Salk worried over the safety of a live polio vaccine – how astute, how correct, how prophetic?

IPV, a vaccine born breaking all conventions and rituals of scientists was not acceptable in the family of conservative aristocrats. The proletariat and developing countries had to be protected from such a perverse product. If they suffer torment as a result, so be it – they can thank the scientists and public health leaders for getting to them the legitimate vaccine, OPV. Torment there was – in 1962, the year after introducing OPV in the USA, 24 children came down with vaccine-caused polio. IPV was, on the other hand, completely safe.

True, OPV was a fascinating vaccine, given as oral drops, avoiding the needle, and inexpensive to manufacture. All good points. One could debate if polio eradication would have come on the global health agenda if OPV had not been available. Maybe, maybe not.

One could also speculate that in the absence of a live vaccine, with the availability of completely safe and exquisitely effective IPV and completely safe and exquisitely effective measles vaccine, both given by injection and both embraced by routine immunization programmes the world over, polio and measles might have been chosen for simultaneous eradication by global health leaders.

In that case, without the distractions brought in by OPV, polio and measles together could have been eradicated decades ago. Global history of disease eradication might have been quite different. Speculations are only speculations – they do not answer questions factually. However, between measles and polio, public health experts would have given higher priority for measles eradication since measles killed about the same number of children as polio paralysed.[2] Therefore the speculation, that in a world without OPV, the history of polio eradication might have been very different, is within the realm of high probability.

OPV was not a very safe vaccine – vaccine-caused polio in the vaccinated and in contacts was obvious, unmistakable. But, there was another more sinister possibility – that vaccine viruses would spread and also could regain virulence. What was its 'worst case' potential? Well, viruses derived from the vaccine could replace wild viruses. When would such a problem become serious? Well, when the universally high prevalence of immunity induced by wild polioviruses decline, the vaccine viruses could take advantage and exhibit their ugly face. Is that not exactly what has happened? From the year 2000, that ugly face of vaccine viruses has appeared in too many places too often. Since 2000 such viruses are called vaccine-derived. They cause outbreaks of polio.

The top scientists and public health leaders failed to read the early signals of this sinister safety problem. They failed in their prophetic role. They saw the signals but failed to interpret their meaning. Scientists ought to observe with open eyes (to see everything, not cherry-picking information and evidence) and interpret with closed eyes (analytically, unbiased, all possibilities considered). Observation is nothing; interpretation is everything.

Cutter incident

Adding fuel to the fire of dismay of traditional polio scientists, who believed in live vaccine, now watching the success of IPV, was the unfortunate Cutter incident. There were reports of children developing polio soon after receiving IPV manufactured by Cutter Laboratories in Berkeley, California. This tragic incident had resulted in 200 children with polio paralysis and ten deaths.[3] Investigations later revealed that the culprit was the residual live virus in the hastily released vaccines without completing and passing the crucial step of safety check-in monkeys. Unknown to many, the safety test had been done in monkeys, and it had failed, and that information was ignored and suppressed by those who should have known better. The action that was necessary, to withhold Cutter vaccine until investigated, was not taken.

That was a silly but serious human error -- a scientist in the National Institutes of Health had actually detected that the Cutter vaccine was not completely inactivated before it was released.[4] We quote from the book, The Health Century; *"It is little known that NIH's Laboratory of Biologics Control, which had certified the Salk vaccine, had received advance warning of problems. And that warning came from its staff microbiologist, Dr Bernice Eddy"*. She had reported to her superiors that the vaccine lot from Cutter had paralysed monkeys inoculated with it. She reported it to the then Director of NIH, who ignored the information. Quoting Bernice Eddy: "*They went ahead and released the vaccine anyway, a lot of it. The monkeys they just disregarded.*" (Ibid, p 69). Cutter incident could and should have been averted. How the human mind works to makes decisions is not always edifying.

Using the lesson from the Cutter incident, all IPV made ever since had been completely safe. The Cutter Company did not survive the 'scandal'.

About the 'full circle' of IPV

IPV was very popular in the USA at first, for a few years, then it lost (lost, passively -- is not the right word; removed, actively -- is more appropriate) its popularity, and was abandoned, but now it has regained acceptance and popularity in the USA since the year 1996, coming a full circle. The full circle has much drama that needs to be reported, repeated.

The drama describes the behaviour of powerful leaders who make decisions for people and nations, based on their discretion and judgment. We trust their judgment, believing that all aspects had been considered. Occasionally we get disappointed, disillusioned.

In personality development courses, teachers emphasize that decisions should not be made when emotionally disturbed – either in euphoria, anger, dejection, despair or hatred. These emotions make people biased, even prejudiced. Or else they become unrealistically generous. We must self-examine our mood when we make important decisions. We show that abandoning IPV was based on hatred, hence highly problematic in public health.

Returning to IPV was undoubtedly the correct choice in the US, pragmatic and ethical, as soon as the safety problems of OPV were detected, documented.

If IPV is the vaccine of choice since 1999, had it not always been the vaccine of choice? Nothing had changed with the vaccine since the mid-1980s to make any difference in the choice. Nothing had changed in the biology of wild polioviruses. In 2000 the target year of global polio eradication had arrived, but some 30-odd countries still had wild virus polio prevalent in them. The reason for the USA to shift policy back to IPV was that the polio paralysis in OPV-given children, caused by vaccine viruses, was also polio and that too entirely avoidable.

While the WHO had not defined what exactly polio eradication was, the Vellore school had defined it as "zero incidence of poliovirus infection, wild and vaccine".

For 30 years, the USA had used OPV exclusively –every year facing 8-10 children with VAPP and compensating them with about 3 million dollars per child. In case the Vellore school's definition got wider acceptance, the USA could not be assessed polio eliminated after the due date, 2000. The decision to switch from OPV to IPV was probably based on belated compulsions of compassion and ethics – the timing was most probably to comply with the clear definition demanding zero infection with vaccine viruses.

The USA story provides the only way forward for the polio eradication program – a transition from OPV to IPV must be achieved expeditiously – if eradication is the real goal. More on that in the chapter on the Way Forward.

The year 2000 provided a clear and strong signal, unmistakable – unless you observed with closed eyes and interpreted with open eyes. There are many ways to 'skin a cat' – the eradication program ought to have accepted the full circle reality and put a stop to all polio caused by vaccine viruses and vaccine-derived viruses the fastest possible way.

That was the true lesson USA taught the world, through Salk, O'Connor and Thomas Francis in the 1950s and the policy leaders of the 1990s. Polio is the enemy, not Salk vaccine, not the 'public'.

Jonas Salk and Influenza vaccine

Some critics have suggested that IPV was developed by Salk by a fluke. We feel it was the outcome of new thinking – a new understanding of immunology. The circumstantial evidence comes from the influenza vaccine– another virus infection, that too on the respiratory tract mucosal surface, for which the most popular vaccine is a killed or inactivated virus vaccine.

The inactivated influenza virus vaccine was the 'brain child' of Jonas Salk. Influenza virus infection is on the upper respiratory mucosa. Poliovirus infection begins in the throat mucosa and then moves onto intestinal mucosa. During the time Salk was beginning to experiment with vaccines against these two mucosal infections, the general belief among all virologists was that live attenuated virus vaccines were necessary to protect against such viral diseases. Salk ideated otherwise, and both the inactivated influenza virus vaccine and the inactivated poliovirus vaccine were born out of his logic and experiments.

In 1934, Jonas Salk, 19 years old, joined the University and Bellevue Hospital Medical College, soon renamed New York University College of Medicine. Ten years earlier, Albert Sabin had graduated from the same Medical College.

The first year started with classes in Anatomy, Physiology and Biochemistry. After one class test in Biochemistry, Professor Keith Cannan asked Jonas Salk to see him in his office. What the professor said was that he appreciated Jonas's analysis of a question in the test that had no correct answer.

Would Salk take one year off, accept a fellowship with a stipend, help Cannan in his research, and teach Biochemistry? This episode gives the picture of an unusual medical student – an erudite logical thinker. Both the stipend and the chance to do some research persuaded him to take one year off medical studies and work under Cannan.

One project entailed culturing streptococci (bacteria causing sore throat and tonsillitis), concentrating the bacteria by centrifugation over a long time, and inoculating the sedimented bacteria into rabbits. The purpose was to induce antibodies. The centrifuge was small, and he had to run the machine over and over again to handle a large volume of bacterial culture fluid. Salk thought of a method to get the bacteria to clump together for easy harvest. Through trial and error, (more by error) he discovered that a small amount of calcium phosphate would do the trick. That was a breakthrough, by fluke, if you like.

What happened was: Salk was trying to make bacteria clump by freezing the culture fluid. He used ice with calcium phosphate (to lower the melting point, just as ice cream was made in olden days using sodium chloride to delay the melting of ice). That did not work, but one time a little calcium chloride leaked into the culture fluid, and the bacteria clumped.

Sheer serendipity, but also astute observation, open eyes, open mind -- typical of Jonas Salk. Bacteriologists were now able to separate bacteria from large volumes of culture fluid, saving much time and effort. This simple but elegant method and many experimental results were published in the prestigious *Proceedings of the Society of Experimental and Biological Medicine*, in 1936, when Jonas was 21 years and doing pre-clinical courses in a medical college.

In 1936 Salk was back in the medical college – for lectures and clinical postings. In one lecture, he heard that killed bacteria could be used as a vaccine since they induced antibody response. Tetanus and diphtheria could be prevented by vaccination, vaccines made through another approach – the vaccine made from tetanus and diphtheria toxins, rendering them non-toxic by chemical treatment. In the next lecture, it was said that vaccines against virus diseases had to be live attenuated, not killed or inactivated. The two viral vaccines – smallpox vaccine showed by Edward Jenner to protect against smallpox, and rabies vaccine developed by Louis Pasteur through laboratory adaptation and manipulation for attenuation of the rabies virus, were both live virus vaccines. In 1936 a yellow fever vaccine was being tested in Brazil – Max Theiler developed it through a similar process – laboratory adaptation and manipulation for attenuation of yellow fever virus.

The pattern was set. The pattern became dogma --live attenuated viruses were necessary to protect against viral diseases. Science opposes the very idea of dogma. But many scientists do not understand.

Salk thought that if the human immune system would respond to non-infectious killed bacteria and even tetanus and diphtheria toxoids that are simpler proteins, it should also respond to inactivated viruses in a vaccine. He asked the professor why killed viruses could not make a vaccine. The professor said *"Not knowing why it's true, isn't the same as it being untrue"*.[5] Salk grabbed the first opportunity to test his question for a scientific answer, as we will see in a minute.

In 1939, Salk was in his final year in medical college. The same year there was a new head of the Department of Bacteriology in the New York University Medical College. He was Thomas Francis Jr. He had come from the prestigious Rockefeller Institute and had to his credit the discovery of an influenza virus different from the one already known. Jonas Salk requested Tom Francis for an opportunity to test his hypothesis that killed virus would induce antibody response.[6]

Francis had already worked with experimental influenza virus infection in laboratory mice. He allowed Salk to experiment – to inoculate mice with a killed virus, grown in mouse lung, killed with ultraviolet light, inject in fresh mice and measure antibody response. Salk worked in the medical college laboratory under Francis for all the mouse work, and in the Rockefeller Institute to inactivate the virus under UV light. By the time Jonas Salk graduated in the medical college, he had answered his question – the killed virus was sufficient, nay, efficient to induce influenza virus antibodies.

The dogma that a live attenuated vaccine was necessary to protect against viral diseases was not yet proven wrong with this one discovery. There was no proof that antibody would protect against influenza. Here is a mucosal infection, not a systemic infection. Influenza viruses do not invade tissues. So protection is needed on the mucosal surface. Would an inactivated virus vaccine provide protection on mucosal surfaces, not merely systemic antibody?

That was a big question if one wanted to make a killed virus influenza vaccine. That would have a bearing on Salk's future studies on polio, another virus infection on mucosal surfaces that also goes systemic as body tissues are invaded.

Salk did get an opportunity to test it out in just a few years. The result of his research actually changed the world. Influenza is surely a surface infection – the virus does not enter the bloodstream. So, one could not equate antibody response with protection from disease. Will a killed virus vaccine protect or not?

This information was invaluable to Thomas Francis, who was appointed in 1941 as the Director of the Commission on Influenza of the Armed Forces Epidemiological Board. The Second World War was raging in Europe. American soldiers were deployed in large numbers in Europe. Because of the urgency of the need to protect American soldiers from influenza, the regulatory agency fast-tracked the safety and efficacy testing of the 'Salk-Francis' killed virus influenza vaccine in American troops. By now influenza viruses were grown in hens' eggs, and large volumes of the virus could be harvested from infected egg fluids. And who did the laboratory work followed by the fieldwork?

Jonas Salk, age 27 years, a relatively unknown researcher of virology. And who got all the credit? Thomas Francis Jr, 41 years and a well-known medical scientist and virologist known for his influenza work. You have got to be somebody before anybody gives you credit for your achievement. If not, your boss in the department where you work will be assigned credit for what was done in his/her department, under 'supervision and guidance'.

Thomas Francis Jr. had worked as a scientist-researcher in the famous Rockefeller Institute in New York, where he had isolated influenza virus, the first in the USA, repeating the work of British scientists who had already isolated a few strains of influenza virus. Francis had also isolated an influenza virus that was different from all earlier isolates. Later Francis was Professor and Head of the Bacteriology Department in the New York University College of Medicine, where Jonas Salk was a medical student and intern while Francis was already head of a teaching-cum-research department.

In 1941 Francis moved to the School of Public Health, University of Michigan, Ann Arbor, Michigan. In the University's Medical College, Francis had a joint appointment as Paediatric Faculty. After medical graduation, Jonas Salk joined Francis in 1941 and continued his research on influenza vaccine under him.

Salk has not been accused by anybody of claiming credit for his work on influenza vaccine in any public forum. In fact, hardly anybody knows that the killed influenza virus vaccine used universally was the brainchild of Jonas Salk. He was not a publicity seeker as he had been accused by jealous contemporaries with regard to 'Salk vaccine'. Salk always called it the killed virus vaccine – it was the popular media that gave the vaccine the name Salk vaccine.

IPV brought bad name for Jonas Salk

In 1947, at age 33, Jonas Salk decided to work independently. He left Thomas Francis's department and joined the University of Pittsburg in Pennsylvania State. He was in need of funds to develop the Microbiology Department. Good fortune smiled on him in Pittsburg. The National Foundation for Infantile Paralysis was looking for laboratories to work on polioviruses, with a promise of liberal funding. Jonas Salk had applied, apparently for getting funds for his department, and was successful.

By 1948, three separate antigenic types (or serotypes) of polioviruses had been identified. The National Foundation for Infantile Paralysis (NFIP) wanted to check if there were more serotypes or not – if a vaccine is ever made, it should contain all serotypes – therefore that information was very important. Notice, NFIP (read Basil O'Connor) was already thinking of a vaccine.

The prescribed work would have been tedious, time-consuming and not intellectually challenging. NFIP had collected a large number of poliovirus isolates, and they were divided among four laboratories. At that time the tests had to be done in monkeys since no other established method was available for typing the poliovirus isolates. Monkeys had to be infected with selected types of polioviruses, and after recovery, they had to be challenged with unknown types and see if the animals got sick. If they did not, it was the same type as previously inoculated.

Every new virus had to be checked against three types. Monkeys were expensive to purchase, and the project was quite expensive. In 1949, polioviruses were shown to grow in laboratory maintained cell culture. John Enders, Thomas

Weller and Frederick Robinson working in Boston, had shared the 1954 Nobel Prize for this work.

Quoting from the book 'Polio: An American Story' by Oshinsky DM: *"When the official word came from Stockholm, Enders made it clear that he would accept the honour only as part of a team that included his junior colleagues, Robbins and Weller. In doing so, he set a standard for generosity against which future researchers, Jonas Salk in particular, would be judged -- and found wanting."* [7] Judged, all right – but very unfair -- prejudiced or ill-informed or both?

Enders was simply honest, not generous. Gifting undeserved credit, such as the authorship of papers, to colleagues, is looked down upon by scientists. No one can gift Nobel Prize: if Enders named his junior colleagues to share the honour, the reason had to be legitimate, generosity excluded. Enders, Weller and Robbins had worked as a team. Their studies were focused on chickenpox – trying to grow chickenpox virus in human fetal skin and muscle tissue culture. One day Thomas Weller suggested to Enders if they could try putting some poliovirus (already available in the freezer) into the tissue culture.[8] Enders gave the go-ahead. The poliovirus strain they had in Harvard was called Lansing, different from the one in Rockefeller Institute that would not grow in non-neural tissue culture. The virus was put in, and a few days later, the fluid was inoculated in monkeys, and they got polio. Enders looked at the cells under the microscope – the cells looked sick and swollen. They then grew poliovirus in kidney cell in culture – human foetal kidney and monkey kidney. No honest scientist would have accepted credit without sharing with the team for the work they did together, particularly when the very idea had come from one of them. That situation was specific for that occasion.

Jonas Salk's situation was entirely different. He swam alone against current; he was alone in his anti-dogma pursuit. Sure, he had hired medical and technical staff, some of them very competent, but, the idea and the effort of creating a killed virus preparation and giving it to animals first (with help from technicians) and humans next (he did that himself) was to Salk's credit. Salk was not awarded the Nobel Prize. The only major recognition Salk got was the President's Medal. That was for the individual; sharing was out of the question.

What about Sabin? Essentially one-man research, very much like Salk's. Was Sabin ever weighed against Enders by anyone? We are using this vignette to illustrate the prejudice and antipathy against the man Salk for which reason the vaccine bearing his name was discredited in the USA – without any worry that the very process was the 'cause' of polio in hundreds of thousands of children worldwide. Its echoes have not died out yet. Devils hide in details.

There is a small book by Robert Greene; "The Concise 48 Laws of Power."[9] Law No. 38 is stated in this book as *"Think as you like, but behave like others"*.

The opening paragraph is titled "Judgment". We quote*: "If you make a show of going against the times, flaunting your unconventional ideas and unorthodox ways, people will think you only want attention and that you look down upon them. They will find a way to punish you for making them feel inferior. It is far safer to blend in and nurture the common touch. Share your originality only with tolerant friends and those who are sure to appreciate your uniqueness."*

Dr Jonas Salk is presented as an illustration of the above lesson. We quote: *"Do not be so foolish as to imagine that in our own time the old orthodoxies are gone. Jonas Salk, for instance, thought that science had gotten past politics and protocol. And so, in his search for a polio vaccine, he broke all the rules – going public with discovery before showing it to the scientific community, taking credit for the vaccine without acknowledging the scientists who had paved the way, making himself a star.*

The public may have loved him, but scientists shunned him. His disrespect for his community's orthodoxies left him isolated, and he wasted years trying to heal the breach and struggling for funding and cooperation."

All right, the public loved him, scientists shunned him; did they also conflate him with the vaccine named after him? Scientists, if they were true followers of science, would surely have been honest and objective about the vaccine even if it bore the name of its developer whom they shunned.

Salk had sought help from Enders for poliovirus in cell culture only if Enders himself was not working on a polio vaccine. Help was denied in spite of the fact that Enders himself was not interested in developing a vaccine against polio. So Salk learned tissue culture methods by himself.

In 1949 and thereafter, Jonas Salk grew poliovirus in test tubes and bottles in which monkey kidney cells were grown, and induced antibodies in laboratory animals by injecting them with killed polioviruses. Thus he made antibodies to the three known poliovirus types and using the antibodies clinched the fact that all strains of polioviruses supplied by the NFIP belonged to just the three types. A vaccine needed only three types represented.

Beginning in 1949, Salk began working on a vaccine based on his logic that a killed virus vaccine, like that against influenza, would be a very safe vaccine, if found effective. He already had viruses growing in cell cultures – so large volumes were already in hand to develop a vaccine. He already had developed a method to kill the virus without losing its ability to induce antibody. The proof of principle of a killed virus vaccine was already in hand.

Manhattan Project and Project Polio Vaccine

In 1941, Japan attacked Pearl Harbour, a US Naval Base in Hawaii – on 7 December Pearl harbour was bombed. That made President Franklin D Roosevelt decide to join World

War II, aligning with Great Britain, France and Russia. On 28 December 1942, Roosevelt ordered the formation of the 'Manhattan Project' essentially to create the atomic bomb. On August 6 and 10, 1945, US bombed Hiroshima and Nagasaki – Japan surrendered on 14 August.[10]

Basil O'Connor would certainly have been fully aware of the dramatic developments that led to the formation of the Manhattan Project and its success. A large number of scientists had worked in several laboratories, under the leadership of J Robert Oppenheimer. Science was the vehicle, scientists were the players, but all rituals of science were suspended for a greater cause than the advancement of science -- the sole goal being the bomb using nuclear fission of uranium and plutonium.

It is naïve to think that Basil O'Connor was not influenced or inspired by the Manhattan Project as he was himself engaged in another war – the war on polio.

There is no direct evidence. Most probably he understood the difference between letting scientists follow their noses and come up with solutions to problems in their own sweet time, or commission research with a specific goal given top priority. O'Connor's actions, serially several of them, fit with this latter proposition. A vaccine became his single-minded goal as the results of scientific studies pointed to its potential, for achieving which in the shortest time, all rituals of science had to be suspended.

Two rival vaccines against one disease, polio

It is hard to imagine that serious thought, to make a polio vaccine -- imitating the Manhattan Project -- but not telling anyone, except perhaps Jonas Salk -- had not crossed O'Connor's mind. We guess also that Salk was probably privy to the Project Polio Vaccine concept of O'Connor. Those five years, 1949 to 1954, were perhaps the most trying time for Salk, unlike any other scientist who was not commissioned for a specific goal. Why else would a highly successful scientist suddenly retire from science – the moment mission was accomplished? Sure, this is speculation, but read the whole story.

Let us search for insights regarding the relationship between Roosevelt and O'Connor. In 1933 Roosevelt became US President. *"Basil O'Connor wrote all or part of many of Roosevelt's early speeches, including his acceptance speech for the presidential nomination in 1932. He helped recruit academic advisors for the Brain Trust and business leaders for the Cabinet, served as personal lawyer to the Roosevelt family, organised Roosevelt's papers into what would eventually become the first presidential library, and continue to be one of the most reliable contributors to Roosevelt's many campaigns."1*

*"Roosevelt trusted O'Connor as he did few others, and brought him into the inner chambers of power – a heady position that never kept O'Connor from following his own policies and interest, even when they disagreed with the president's"*1 In 1937 Roosevelt established the National Foundation for Infantile Paralysis at the behest of O'Connor. From then on, O'Connor's major attention was on the fight against polio. O'Connor had the special knack of keeping some thoughts, events and actions to himself.

Scientists pride themselves with curiosity motive for research. Those who work for scientists are technicians. When Jonas Salk agreed to undertake the typing of poliovirus isolates, senior polio scientists misread Salk – that he was willing to do boring, repetitive tests and that he was not a curiosity-driven scientist, but a technician at heart. Salk was raising funds for establishing a department, with competent technical hands, for future studies. He had to familiarise with polioviruses, and he achieved his immediate goals elegantly – he learned all about polioviruses, and he got liberally funded.

He needed a lot of funds. And the National Foundation for Infantile Paralysis needed an Oppenheimer-like polio scientist – but no established polio scientist would play ball. Salk was nurtured by NFIP to become the Oppenheimer of the polio vaccine. He did just that.

Louis Pasteur had made a live attenuated rabies virus vaccine grown in rabbit spinal cords. In the 1880s, viruses were not known; so we are doing a time-machine trick putting new knowledge in old context. Fourteen doses of emulsified rabbit spinal cords infected with the laboratory-adapted rabies virus had to be given on serial days. The oldest spinal cord, air-dried in clean laboratory air, contained some live and a lot of inactivated viruses. The earlier ones contained increasing doses of live viruses until the one-day-old spinal cord contained nearly all live viruses. David Semple, a British Army medical officer showed in 1912 that the same laboratory-adapted and attenuated rabies virus could be grown in rabbit brain or sheep brain, and chemically inactivate the virus content, and yet it induced antibodies – thus the Pasteur live rabies virus vaccine was replaced by the Pasteur-Semple inactivated rabies virus vaccine. Thus, Jonas Salk was not the first to create a killed virus vaccine.

Jonas Salk showed the same principle with the influenza virus. Rabies is a 'systemic' infection, and it is obvious that the antibody would protect the person while the rabies virus is between the site of the bite and the nervous tissue.

IPV was the first of the two vaccines developed against polio. IPV was licensed for commercial production in the USA in 1955. When the oral poliovirus vaccine (OPV) was developed and became available (licensed in the USA in 1961 but increasingly used only during 1964-68), there were two vaccines against polio, with contrasting, hence potentially complementary, properties.

That was a unique situation, hugely advantageous situation, one that offered the potential of eradication of polio, provided policymakers and public health leaders made wise decisions devoid of emotion, biases and prejudices. Sadly, things did not go right.

In the country of origin of the two vaccines, namely USA, OPV became popular and IPV unpopular after obtaining maximum benefit from IPV over 12-13 years – some 98-99% reduction of the burden of polio. The vaccines were not rivals – they were made to look like rivals by powerful people.

Time is a great healer, evidence wins over faith

In 1968, thirteen years after IPV's introduction, the USA adopted an exclusive OPV policy. Then in 1999, thirty-one years later, in a complete *volte facie,* USA rejected OPV and adopted an exclusive IPV policy. By then nearly 300 children had developed vaccine-associated paralytic polio, VAPP. If the public worshipped Salk, the scientists taught the public a lesson.

The year 2000 was the target year of global polio eradication. The Vellore school had defined polio eradication as reaching zero poliovirus infection, wild and vaccine. USA had about 8-10 cases of VAPP per year until IPV was re-introduced. The WHO had an un-articulated definition of zero infection with wild polioviruses – vaccine-induced polio was the supposedly legitimate price for eradicating wild polioviruses.

Either as pure coincidence or as a wise move of accepting the Vellore definition of polio eradication, in the year 2000 USA managed to truly eliminate polio, including vaccine poliovirus infection, and reach zero polio status. Since then (and only since then) USA has remained totally polio-free, thereby demonstrating that IPV is essential for polio elimination and that continued use of OPV is not compatible with polio elimination. These lessons provided a model for global polio eradication. That was in the year 2000.

Albert Sabin did not just develop a vaccine, OPV, but he created a 'religion' with dogmas, rules and rituals. IPV, its use and its supporters, remained within science – evidence-based. OPV had its champions – IPV needed none. They were not like two science schools – in science, hard facts and evidence are needed, but in religion, deep faith and a large supporting group of believers are good enough.

Some years later, when the live attenuated oral poliovirus vaccine (OPV) against the same disease was developed by Albert Sabin, it could not be tested in a vaccine trial in the US. Such a vaccine trial could only have been designed as a comparison with the already licensed vaccine. So, even without a comparative evaluation, OPV replaced IPV in the US, by Government policy. We have not come across any book on the story of Sabin and OPV. There is one book that describes the history of both vaccines: "An American Story".[7]

The allergy of American biomedical leaders of the 1960s and thereafter, to the Salk vaccine, by which it was rejected from favour, was mainly because they hated the maker of that vaccine. That does not make sense because the scientific assessment of the safety and efficacy of a vaccine and comparison with another vaccine against the same disease, namely OPV, should have been based on objective evidence and not on the personalities involved. It makes some sense only when we learn the background and history of the making of IPV that reads almost like fiction. The twists and turns of that story had collateral victims in top government positions. Many of them – polio experts and policymakers, could retaliate only by rejecting his vaccine.

Although the vaccine was popularly called the Salk vaccine, particularly by the media, it was truly a people's vaccine. The public had funded his research through a private Foundation. Salk never called it the Salk vaccine. By rejecting the vaccine Salk's reputation was dented all right, but the collateral damage that resulted from rejecting IPV and replacing it with OPV was suffered by the public – annually 8-10 children who developed the very disease that IPV would have prevented. Innocent children in unsuspecting families in even larger numbers continue to this day to be victims of polio, victims of the policy that was born out of hatred, and not out of science or compassion.

Scientists and policy-makers are also human

Scientists and powerful policymakers are also humans and vulnerable to human weaknesses of biases and prejudices, even when their determined stand, said to be with good intentions, results in unnecessary human suffering. In politics and its hobby of military actions, often decisions are made for reasons that are not necessarily honourable and not always presented to the public honestly. In science, this problem is not expected to happen since science is by definition, the pursuit of truth. The story of the Salk vaccine became 'complexified' by the 'politics' of its time. Humanity was on the back burner.

Often, when a mistake stares them in the face, leaders tend to argue to prove their decision was no error; that was the best decision. The rejection of the Salk vaccine in the USA was one such erroneous decision. The year after OPV was licensed in the US, 24 children developed polio caused by the live vaccine virus. The vaccine was not fully attenuated. A reversal of decision was the right thing to do until the safety of the vaccine was made acceptable by way of attempts at more attenuation. Yet, those who made that decision defended their decision and did not worry one bit about its ethical dimension.

They went even further, to get a national policy to in favour of OPV in 1964-65. By then polio had been decimated in the US by 99%. Punishing Salk was one thing; punishing the public was unethical. Even if the policymakers and scientists thought that the live attenuated oral vaccine had some advantages over IPV, the proper step would have been to give a choice to the pediatricians and the parents to choose between the two. That was precisely what was done in France. Some other factor or factors played in the USA – no one seems to have pinpointed that factor or those factors.

Bias and prejudice are mostly in the subconscious, and as such, not perceived by the owner of the mind who perceives mostly through the cognitive domain. Biases and prejudices are mostly in the affective, subjective or emotional domain of the mind, not in the objective, intellectual or cognitive domain. Like others, scientists also 'know' some 'facts' by logical conclusion and know other so-called 'facts' by belief. Many of us, humans, do not differentiate between the knowledge of the cognitive realm and knowledge of the faith realm. It is strange that the belief that Salk was not a good and proper scientist, but a selfish attention seeker, led, we suspect, to the associated belief that his vaccine was not a proper scientific product. This negative approach to the Salk vaccine has taken several forms; the most relevant for us is that it is not considered a 'complete' vaccine for community use. It 'only' protects the vaccinated children, not the neighbours. But it does protect all vaccinated children – which is the function of a good vaccine. We will come back to this later.

True, the public adored him; but scientists shunned him. But, wait a minute; he did not go public with his discovery. That is not corroborated by historical facts. Salk did not claim any credit, but credit was thrust upon him. The inactivated polio vaccine was his idea, one that was unconventional and original. No one else deserves credit for it – as we will show presently. One man, a powerful man at that, Basil O'Conner, the Director of the private Foundation – National Foundation for Infantile Paralysis, the agency that had funded all of Salk's research, took ownership of Salk's experimental vaccine and independently organised a massive vaccine trial.

The vaccine trial was not Salk's idea – Salk indeed was kept out of the planning and execution of the trial. Salk did not put down other polio scientists – if they felt inferiority in any manner, that might have been tinged with jealousy also – after all, there were many senior polio scientists working towards a polio vaccine, but this 'upstart' polio researcher outsmarted all of them and came up with a safe and effective polio vaccine, within five years of initiation into polio research. Call him underdog or dark horse, but he made a world record.

No one else had paved the way for Salk to get the idea of an inactivated virus vaccine. Basil O'Conner saw the merit and potential in Salk's research product. And he was a lawyer, not swayed by the belief system of virologists who maintained that only a live attenuated virus vaccine would be fully effective as protective against a virus disease – here, polio.

In fact, Salk is the one who created the inactivated influenza vaccine that we all continue to use – but he never craved for getting credit for his work on influenza. After rejecting the Salk polio vaccine, people have found many false reasons why the vaccine had to be rejected. The only reason was anger, an emotional reason, nothing to do with science or facts. Rejecting the Salk vaccine had created many problems in polio prevention, control, elimination and eradication as we point out different ways.

Summation

The story of the development, massive clinical trial and registration of the inactivated poliovirus vaccine in record short time, has a fictional flavour – Jonas Salk its undisputed hero. The National Foundation for Infantile Paralysis was established in 1938, in response to recurrent polio outbreaks in the USA, by President Franklin D Roosevelt, himself a victim of polio paralysis below the waist. His Law Partner Basel O'Connor managed the affairs of NFIP and raised funds and wisely spent it on vaccine development. Salk, funded by NFIP, wanted a safe vaccine for which he created the inactivated poliovirus vaccine, IPV. O'Connor manoeuvred the vaccine research until IPV was field tested, registered and distributed freely to all children, thereby conquering polio in the US. Unfortunately, polio scientists and public health leaders, all conventional thinkers, disliked the unconventional way the polio problem was solved. Salk became a public hero, but also target of hatred by the scientific establishment. As a result USA formally rejected IPV after getting the best benefit from it for over a decade, and replaced it with the live attenuated oral poliovirus vaccine OPV. What Salk feared was that a live virus vaccine may not be completely safe. He was right, but his vaccine was kept out of the USA until 1996, after which it was re-introduced in the US and all OPV withdrawn from 1999, precisely for its safety problems. Countries that use IPV exclusively do not have any polio. The echoes of the dislike for Salk have not died out in the global polio eradication program that continues without accepting its preeminent role to complete and conclude the program.

5. ALBERT SABIN AND ORAL POLIOVIRUS VACCINE

"No science is immune to the infection of politics and the corruption of power" Jacob Bronowski

Dr Albert Sabin had a head start of some 17-18 years over Dr Jonas Salk in polio research.[1] Both had graduated in Medicine, with MD degree, from the New York University College of Medicine (previously called University and Bellevue Hospital Medical College) – Sabin in 1931 and Salk in 1940. Sabin straightaway began working on polio – in the famous Rockefeller Institute. Although Sabin is best known for his work on polio, he had worked on many other problems, many with great success. He was the recipient of over 40 honorary degrees from various universities.

A breakthrough in polio virology, with an unfortunate twist

In 1936 he had a breakthrough: Sabin and senior research colleague Dr Olitsky successfully grew a strain of poliovirus in human embryonic brain tissue cultured in laboratory ware.[2] In those days poliovirus was studied in experimental animals, mostly monkeys and chimpanzees. So, growing poliovirus in the laboratory was a breakthrough.

Sabin and Olitsky had no success in growing poliovirus in non-neural tissues *in vitro* in the laboratory and concluded that poliovirus grew only in nervous system tissues. At that time, Jonas Salk was still in medical college and was working on inactivated influenza virus vaccine under Professor of Bacteriology Dr Thomas Francis Jr who had by then shifted from The Rockefeller Institute to the New York University Medical College.

Those days, culturing tissue in laboratory ware (*in vitro* or more exactly *ex-vivo*) itself was a cumbersome procedure – it was not like modern cell culture – but tiny bits of tissue kept alive in a culture medium. Today's cell culture is a layer of cells, growing as a sheet on glass or plastic surface.

The Rockefeller strain of poliovirus was a peculiar one, adapted to the monkey nervous system, and non-representative of natural polioviruses. The Rockefeller strain did not grow in non-neural tissue. In 1936 poliovirus was believed to be one single entity; the fact that there were three distinct types was unknown.

In 1949 Enders, Weller and Robbins reported growing poliovirus in laboratory cultures of non-neural tissue of human embryonic origin, for which discovery they got the Nobel Prize.[3] If Sabin had tried another strain of poliovirus, not the one in Rockefeller Institute, he would have proved that it grew in non-neural tissue culture. Would that have won him Nobel Prize? Could such a thought have crossed his mind?

Jonas Salk began his work on polio in 1949. Youngner JS, working in the laboratory of Jonas Salk perfected the method of growing polioviruses in monolayer cultures of monkey kidney cells.[4]

Sabin's attenuated virus strains were ready in 1956

Sabin had been thinking of a live attenuated poliovirus vaccine for a long time. He needed an *in vitro* system to grow large amounts of polioviruses in order to manipulate and attenuate them into a vaccine. We do not know why he did not pursue his tissue culture work even after knowing polioviruses had three serotypes. He did not seem to be in any hurry.

The possibility of growing large amounts of polioviruses in the laboratory opened up by 1950s, thanks to Enders, Weller, Robbins. Salk and Youngner were successful with their monolayer cell culture system of monkey kidney cells. Here, Salk had a head start of one year over Sabin. Salk had already learned to inactivate polioviruses grown in cell cultures – so he could move fast to make a candidate vaccine that could be tested in laboratory animals, including monkeys, and then move into humans. That he accomplished in just 4 years; a candidate vaccine including the three types was available in 1954; Salk's inactivated poliovirus vaccine (IPV) was licensed in USA and a few other countries in April 1955. Now Sabin was indeed in a hurry.

Sabin had the firm belief that only a live infectious vaccine that infected the alimentary tract would protect against polio effectively. He had already shown that children with polio had intestinal infection, resulting in copious amounts of poliovirus shed in stools. Showing poliovirus infection on intestinal mucosa was another breakthrough. That reinforced in his mind, that a mucosal vaccine, hence live and infectious, was the right way to protect humans from polio. He wanted to make a live virus vaccine, and make it as safe as he could and as fast as he could.

Sabin was not the first to develop candidate strains of live poliovirus vaccine – but the others had no way of testing for neurovirulence except oral feeding of chimpanzees and monkeys. Oral feeding may not always cause paralysis in them. For comparison, if you feed wild poliovirus type 3 in 1000 children, only one would develop polio paralysis, since the case-to-infection ratio is 1:1000. Safety was not easy to prove.

Herald Cox working in the Lederle company and Hilary Koprowski working in the Wistar Institute had developed what they thought were attenuated strains. In 1950, Koprowski had fed 20 children with his attenuated type 2 strain – that was the very first deliberate feeding of a candidate live poliovirus vaccine.[5]

Safety could not be tested in humans but could be tested in chimpanzees or monkeys. Sabin wanted an objective and quantifiable method of testing for neurovirulence (during those early days, the term used was 'neurotropism' for what we now call neurovirulence), and creating a reproducible test in the monkey was crucial for his progress and eventual success. He would inject the vaccine preparation in the lumbar spinal cords of monkeys and compare the pathology with spinal cords of monkeys injected with wild poliovirus. The pathology could be graded as 0 to 4+.

Sabin's 'monkey neurovirulence test' was key to his success – he could predict which virus preparation was nearly fully attenuated or partially attenuated or not attenuated. That gave him an edge over other investigators working on developing live attenuated poliovirus vaccine. By 1956 Sabin had attenuated strains of all three types of poliovirus – types 1, 2 and 3 – non-neurovirulent in the spinal cord tests.

Competition among these three groups – Sabin, Koprowski and Cox, was acute. Not to give up, Cox through Lederle Company managed to feed a mixture of the three types of their attenuated polioviruses (in other words a trivalent vaccine candidate) to 280,000 persons in Berlin, New Hampshire, in 1960. Twenty-three cases of polio occurred among the vaccinated and 15 more in their contacts. What was most disconcerting was the occurrence of 8 cases in the community without contact with the vaccinated.[6] Cox had no good method to measure the degree of neurovirulence prior to human testing. His virus was transmissible.

Sabin was not to be defeated. He had selected the best-attenuated strains of types 1, 2 and 3 in 1956 and in 1957 gave them orally to his own family members first and then to others. By then polio burden had begun steeply declining in the US and no agency, particularly the NFIP and Basil O'Connor, had no inclination to conduct another trial of a new polio vaccine. Sabin himself could not do a vaccine trial in the USA because children had to be given Salk vaccine; withholding Salk vaccine for a trial of OPV was unethical.

Dr Joseph Melnick, working in Baylor College of Medicine in Houston, Texas, compared the three strains of type 3 in hundreds of monkeys in 1958 and concluded that the Sabin strain was the most attenuated.[7]

Salk's apprehension was very valid. Live vaccine viruses spreading from the vaccinated to the unvaccinated was a big liability – the community-acquired cases with Cox's vaccine were a message that vaccine-virus spread was not good. Would Sabin's attenuated viruses spread from vaccinated children to others? If they did, the safety of such transmitted viruses could not be guaranteed.

Sabin manages to get WHO championing his vaccine

The WHO established an Expert Committee on Poliomyelitis in 1957, after Sabin had fed all three types of his attenuated strains to humans. The Committee met in July 1957.[8] Sabin was on that Committee but not Salk. A bias in favour or Sabin's experimental vaccine over Salk's proven and licensed vaccine was obvious already in 1957, but its reason is not clear. Was it the echo of the hatred of Salk in the USA? Or, was it due to the fascination for an oral vaccine? All other vaccines in current use then were injected. Or was it due to the dogma that only live virus vaccines could protect against virus diseases? If Sabin's influence was the reason to establish that Committee, then Sabin's persuasive arguments were probably the reason for the bias.

The committee *"discussed the vital points involved with the development of live poliovirus vaccines."*[8] The Committee set criteria for selection of vaccine strains – all favoring Sabin's strains. One criterion was: *"Adequate and regular multiplication in the alimentary tract of non-immune human beings should have been demonstrated with [virus] doses in the range of 100,000 median tissue culture infectious dose or less and these infections should be accompanied by an antibody response."*[9]

That criterion was fulfilled in the US; ironically, not in India, Pakistan, Nigeria etc. Even 1,000,000 viruses of type 1 vaccine virus or 300,000 of type 3 did not infect more than 30% of children in South India or more than 10% of children in North India.[10] Strictly speaking Sabin OPV (types 1 and 3) did not fulfil the WHO's own criterion of an acceptable vaccine as far as India and many low income tropical countries were concerned. When this problem was detected and reported, by early 1970s, WHO experts simply did not react.

Sabin vaccine in mass use in USSR

One of the members of the WHO Expert Committee on Poliomyelitis was Dr VD Soloviev from USSR. The next year Sabin supplied his vaccine seed strains to virologists in Moscow and taught them how to grow them up and use as a vaccine. Under the leadership of Dr Chumakov, some 15 million children and young adults were given Sabin vaccine in 1959 and 1960, and the result was an impressive decline of polio.[11]

There were some odd things in their report: for one thing, 3 million persons were given Salk vaccine, the source of which was not mentioned. Did they make IPV by themselves? Was its quality tested? IPV did not reduce the burden of polio in the community, unlike in the USA during 1955 onwards. That information was intriguing. Second, vaccine safety referred only to the usual kinds of adverse reactions common to other injected vaccines, but the paralytic disease was not specially looked for. This study was in stark contrast to the Francis trial of the Salk vaccine, in which both efficacy and safety were carefully monitored. It is not for nothing that the USA is called the Mecca of Public Health.

Polio was highly prevalent in USSR. OPV seemed very effective in preventing polio in the community, particularly when applied on a mass scale. The real adverse reaction to OPV would have been vaccine-polio, indistinguishable from wild-virus polio. Polio in the vaccinated caused by vaccine virus (VAPP) and VAPP in contacts, as well as community-acquired VAPP – all could easily be mistaken for natural polio in spite of vaccination in the vaccinated and natural polio in the unvaccinated. The Russians seemed to have totally missed the reality – they knew OPV was highly effective and assumed it was quite safe also, without evidence.

Those were cold war years – the relationship between USA and USSR was not cordial. When an American vaccine was very popular in the USSR but not in the USA, people felt the irony of the situation. A US emissary visited USSR and reported that the Sabin vaccine was indeed highly efficacious. Largely encouraged by that report, in 1961 Sabin vaccine type 3 was licensed in the USA and was used widely in 1961. In 1962, 24 cases of polio due to type 3 Sabin virus occurred, all proven epidemiologically and/or virologically to be vaccine-related. Strange, but true: the next year Sabin types 2 and 1 were also licensed in the USA. In 1964 trivalent OPV was licensed in the USA. And every year since 1961 there has been a few children with vaccine-polio.

Why did the US not reverse its policy on account of the safety problem of OPV? One would have imagined that a country advocating human rights in all situations would have seen that it was unethical to cause polio in a few while benefitting a large majority. This was especially problematic, as there was an alternate vaccine – IPV -- that was completely safe.

Sabin put forth strong arguments in favor of his vaccine

OPV is a unique vaccine in many ways. It was a 'tricky' vaccine too, as Sabin himself knew – the vaccine viruses infect children, and they shed lots of viruses in their stools over a few weeks – even up to 8 weeks. The viruses that came out in children's stools were more neurovirulent in monkey spinal cord test than the vaccine viruses in the vial.

On both counts – neurovirulence and transmissibility, Sabin's vaccine viruses were not fully attenuated. Virologists have questioned if full attenuation was at all possible with polioviruses. However, Sabin was in a rush to promote his vaccine even as polio had been 'conquered' in the USA by IPV. What Sabin did was to create a dogma to circumvent each problem, in addition to reinforcing an already existing dogma that live virus vaccine was essential against a viral disease.

Sabin's set of dogmas included the following.

Dogma 1. Wild polioviruses enter the child's body through the mouth; therefore, an oral vaccine, given by the 'natural route' was essential for complete immunity, particularly for blocking stool virus shedding. [This was apparently the premise for the strategy of exclusive use of OPV in EPI for polio control and in the program for polio eradication.]

Dogma 2. Sabin's attenuated virus strains constituting OPV was one of the safest of vaccines. It could not and did not ever cause polio. [This is apparently the reason why the eradication program does not count VAPP as polio during the eradication era.]

Dogma 3. When contacts of immunised children were infected by the vaccine viruses, they got free vaccination – a great advantage for OPV – because every child did not need to be vaccinated. [This is apparently still counted as an advantage in spite of knowing that it is morally wrong to let unsuspecting children getting infected with vaccine viruses.]

Dogma 4. A live infectious vaccine, not killed virus vaccine, was necessary to provide long-lasting immunity. With killed vaccine, immune responses will wane, and children will have to be given many repeated doses, while very few doses of OPV will suffice. [This is apparently another reason why exclusive use of OPV was promoted.]

The definition of 'dogma' is: "a principle or principles laid down by an authority and intended to be accepted without question" (Oxford dictionary). Sabin was the world's No. 1 authority as far as poliovirus research was concerned. He had several breakthrough contributions: world's first to grow poliovirus in tissue culture; he disproved that polioviruses entered the brain through the olfactory nerves as claimed by the earlier No 1 authority – Simon Flexner. Sabin had demonstrated that polioviruses infected the intestinal mucosa before causing polio paralysis. He also had developed a test to measure neurovirulence in monkeys.

People love dogmas as they absolve them from taking moral responsibility for actions. Once you believe the authority that created the dogmas, you can trust the dogmas as truth, and need not apply science, do experiments to test the dogmas, and you are assured of being in the company of the like-minded majority. Once dogmas become beliefs, evidence contrary to the beliefs is simply discarded or ignored by the vast majority of believers.

Any dogma could be true – just because it is dogma is no proof that it is not true. But every dogma remains unproven unless checked and proved by science. Sabin's dogmas were apparently accepted by the majority of public health experts who made decisions for the public.

Health Ministry experts in India accepted the dogmas without questioning them. Any dissent was dismissed as motivated.

WHO experts likewise accepted the dogmas without questioning them. The whole edifice of the global polio eradication was built on the sands of these dogmas, not on the rock of scientific evidences.

There is no mystery in the way polio eradication is delayed and has even lost the right path – the very definition of polio eradication could not be clearly stated, apparently blocked by the dogmas. When a definition was proposed like – zero incidence of poliovirus infection, wild and vaccine – it could not be accepted by the believers of the dogmas.

Examining the veracity of the dogmas.

We must take a close look at each of these items to verify if it stands to reason or if it is without evidence or contrary to evidence.

Dogma 1. Wild polioviruses enter the child's body through the mouth and not through the nose. Therefore an oral vaccine is ideal – not a non-infectious vaccine. There is no scientific evidence for oral entry of natural (wild) polioviruses. Epidemiological features favour nasal entry. Dogma remains unproven, most likely incorrect, as described in Chapter 6.

There is no scientific reason that a mucosal live vaccine is essential to protect against disease caused by any mucosal infection. Several vaccines like Human Papilloma Virus vaccine, *Haemophilus influenzae* b vaccine, pneumococcal vaccine, diphtheria vaccine, whooping cough vaccine, typhoid fever vaccine – all non-infectious and injected, against diseases caused by mucosal infections, exhibit very high degree of mucosal protection. IPV is no exception as shown repeatedly in different settings. Belief in dogma remains in spite of overwhelming evidence to the contrary.

Dogma 2. OPV consisting of Sabin's attenuated virus strains was one of the safest of vaccines -- it could not, and did not ever, cause polio. In 3 WHO publications this dogma is repeated: 1976, 1982 and 1988.[10,11,12] There is scientific evidence to the contrary. Dogma had been proven incorrect since 1961, but yet OPV was repeatedly certified as one among the safest of vaccines.

In fact, OPV is the only unsafe vaccine in the current list of some 25 vaccines in regular use under national immunization programmes in many rich countries. No other vaccine under EPI in developing countries (including several new vaccines), causes 'serious adverse reaction' in normal children (and adults), like OPV does. A sign of the psychological effect of the belief in this dogma is that serious-minded and well-meaning polio experts are able to maintain that OPV is one of the safest vaccines.

Dogma 3. When contacts are infected by the vaccine viruses, be happy, they get free vaccination – a great advantage for OPV. Dogma is contrary to both the science of vaccinology and the ethics of biomedical interventions and also ethics of public health.

Nobody has any right to seed a community with potentially polio-causing virus that may get transmitted. Dogma was instrumental in forcing people into acceptance of a risky live virus vaccine.

Dogma 4. A live infectious vaccine was necessary to provide long term immunity; killed virus vaccine cannot induce long term immunity. This has been proven wrong with evidence to the contrary. However, polio experts still hold on to this belief. The longevity of immunity is a function of long-lived plasma cells secreting antibodies and of long-lived memory cells. They can be elicited by live and killed vaccines. IPV elicits long-lasting immunity. Dogma is incorrect. Indeed it takes far fewer numbers of doses of IPV than OPV for inducing robust immunity.

Summation

Creating an attenuated poliovirus vaccine was a heroic and monumental achievement, no doubt. Molecular virology and viral genetics had not been figured out in the 1950s and 1960s. No one can blame Sabin for the fundamental problem of viral genetics that made polioviruses not vulnerable to full attenuation. As single-stranded positive sense RNA virus, minor mutations are extremely common when polioviruses multiply in humans and in cell cultures in the laboratory. Some such mutations made some of the progeny viruses less virulent – and Sabin managed to select out and encourage the less virulent viruses to be concentrated in serial passaging of the viruses in cell cultures. The final versions of viruses, not virulent in monkey spinal cord inoculation test, selected out for vaccine manufacture, were not stable enough in further generations. That was Sabin's dilemma.

The scientific problem was insurmountable; necessary molecular techniques to detect the genes of virulence were not available then. When such techniques became available, ways to delete the genes and yet keep the virus viable were found not practical. Complete attenuation by genetic manipulations make the resultant virus incapable of transmission – such methods are available now by which a novel OPV has been made, but such a vaccine will be a new product that has to go through licensing in all countries that could use them. Too late in the day, for polio eradication.

Sabin then used his persuasive communication skill and convinced contemporary colleagues in science, healthcare and public health that his vaccine viruses were completely attenuated and safe. Sabin's compulsions and motivations are understandable. The uncritical acceptance of Sabin's dogmas by otherwise competent and honest polio experts is difficult to understand. Our explanation puts it in the affective domain of their minds, by which cold, rational, objective evaluation was overlooked and tested-and-found-true evidence was not demanded.

§§§

6. DO WILD POLIOVIRUSES INFECT THROUGH THE NOSE OR THE MOUTH?

When confronted with evidence that is contrary to belief, most people discard evidence and preserve belief.

In the morning, we see the sun rising in the east, moving all day, and setting in the west. The next morning it appears in the east, obviously having completed the circuit. We see the sun going around the earth. But in school, we were taught that it is only an illusion; it is the earth that revolves around the sun – not the other way round. So we have two mutually exclusive paradigms of a geocentric planetary system and heliocentric solar system. You can't blame those who believe what they see and hold on to the model of a geocentric planetary system which counts the sun and moon among all other objects (*'Graha'* in Sanskrit, meaning planets, seven altogether, sun, moon and the five planets visible to the naked eye) that seem to go around the earth. Days of the week are named after these seven.

Teachers are supposed to know everything, so children accept what teachers teach in school. At first, we simply believed what was taught – the paradigm of a heliocentric solar system. With more information, we see that it fits many other phenomena – including solar and lunar eclipses. We can observe various planets moving along roughly the same path as that of the sun, called the ecliptic. The moon also moves near the ecliptic. Planets are seen from the earth as if they are all roughly in one plane, like a disk. The paradigm explains all related phenomena – such as solar and lunar eclipses and waxing and waning of the moon -- all observations fit without anomaly.

For those who believe in the geocentric planetary system, new assumptions are necessary to explain; for example, the eclipses. In the correct paradigm, all observed phenomena fit in. This lesson has relevance in polio eradication, as we will see later on.

In the night, we see the moon revolving around the earth. We were taught in the school that there is no illusion here – we visualise what actually happens. But that does not prove that the sun also revolves around the earth; two virtually identical phenomena, of sun and moon rising in the east and setting in the west, are due to different reasons. One explanation does not fit both observations, seemingly identical. Everything need not be as it seems to be. Observation is nothing; interpretation is everything.

Oddly, why we see the sun going around the earth, resulting in day and night, is for a totally different reason from that of revolution – rotation of the earth around its own axis, completed in 24 hours. Moon also has rotation on its own axis and revolution around the earth. The time taken by the moon for one rotation and one revolution around the earth is identical – that is why moon always presents only one side towards the earth – that is the bright and visible side when the moon reflects sunshine.

Don't we also often show only the bright side to others? Global polio eradication also has its bright and visible side and an invisible dark side that generally remains hidden from the public.

We understand and tend to explain phenomena in paradigms. We tend to believe our paradigms are true. Evidence, contrary to what we believe, tends to create discomfort in mind. That is called cognitive dissonance[1]. The majority of normal people avoid cognitive dissonance by rejecting evidence if it is contrary to belief. Only the exceptional ones double-check to figure out what to accept – paradigm or contrary evidence. The majority hold on to the paradigm – when a threshold number of persons see the evidence as correct, suddenly there is a paradigm shift that the majority then accepts.[2]

Nose or mouth: what difference will that make?

Microbes have two ready-made portals of entry into the human body, the nostrils and the mouth. These are open to the environment. If a virus is in the air, it may be breathed in. If a virus is in water or food, we may ingest it. Which one is the common, natural route of entry of wild polioviruses in order to establish infection in the human host? This question may appear a trivial, as the two portals are very close to each other. On the contrary, this was the most crucial question for consideration when the strategy and tactics were designed for polio eradication.

Think of the two paradigms, one for oral entry (faecal-oral transmission) and the other for nasal entry (respiratory transmission). What is the immediate antecedent source of the virus -- food and water or air? How does the virus get dispersed to reach that source? These are elaborated below. These are needed to complete the paradigm. The correct paradigm will have no anomaly.

The failure of the jumping spider to catch the flies was because of the glass wall between them. Glass in the spider's world view is unknown. The spider was not aware of the barrier. (How do we know this? Evidence is impossible to garner. From its behaviour, we have to surmise and move on.) It believed what it thought it saw – flies landing close by. The spider jumped as it always had done. Without knowing the reason why the flies were not accessible, the spider went on trying again and again. To keep on doing the same thing repeatedly and expecting a different outcome was the spider's problem. Are we not familiar with such situations ourselves, including in the polio eradication efforts?

Nose versus Mouth and the Choice of Vaccine

There are many problems with the eradication efforts such as time over-run; fund-guzzling activities such as the requirement of sophisticated laboratory testing of all poliovirus isolates to determine if they are wild-like, vaccine-like or vaccine-derived, and, the need to search for vaccine-derived viruses in sewage. The program also contravened the equity principle of public health and ethics of immunization. All of them arose as a consequence of the continuing, widespread and exclusive use of OPV without an early realistic 'sunset plan' for OPV to be replaced by IPV. That was the consequence of the belief, without evidence, in the paradigm of faecal-oral transmission -- wild polioviruses entering through the mouth. For that reason, the oral infectious vaccine was assumed (again, without evidence) to be essential.

Oral live vaccine for oral infection by poliovirus sounds logical. Observed facts do not support that view. In fact there is no logic here, only poetic similitude. Typhoid fever is also due to an oral infection (no one disputes that), and small intestine is the first (or primary) site of infection. After that, the infection invades the body tissues and organs and causes disease. The most effective vaccine against typhoid fever is an injected, non-infectious vaccine called 'conjugated Vi vaccine'. Immunity thus induced has a profound effect on the epidemiology of typhoid fever, showing thereby that the disease can be controlled and infection even eliminated if so desired.

Why has a global plan not been developed to eradicate typhoid fever? It is certainly not for want of intervention tools. Typhoid spreads by faecal-oral transmission. Therefore this disease is prevalent only in countries with poor sanitation and hygiene – all of them are low or middle-income countries. They do not have a champion for typhoid eradication. India has an opportunity to lead all developing countries in typhoid elimination, only if India wants to. The bugle call for polio eradication was precisely because it affected all rich countries as much as developing countries. Had it been another disease due to faecal-oral transmission, polio would have been in league with typhoid fever – globally neglected and most unlikely to have been picked for global eradication.

Every infection and its related phenomena of pathology, transmission, as well as the functional efficacy of vaccines against it, are not merely figured out with logic – they have to be observed, interpreted, hypotheses made, tested, verified. That is the scientific approach. Each set for every infectious agent is unique -- a law unto itself. What matters is what is observed and correctly interpreted. Even if polioviruses entered through the mouth (we will argue why that is not the case), infect the intestines and invade into body tissues and organs and cause disease, it does not necessarily mean that an oral infectious vaccine is necessary to protect against polio, control polio or even eliminate polio – unless, of course, there is scientific proof. There is none.

Suppose we let loose vaccine polioviruses into the community. In that case, all polioviruses out there will have to be carefully analysed to see if they are the natural (wild) ones that we want to be eradicated or the introduced ones that we have to live with, as both are polioviruses. Whether public health experts have any right to let loose viruses that can by themselves cause polio, even outbreaks of polio due to cVDPVs, particularly without consent (or even knowledge) of concerned parties, is a question we raise in the chapter on ethics of vaccine-choice and ethics of public health.

If live virus vaccines had been stopped and only IPV was in use, say from before 2000, or about 2000, or soon thereafter, then any poliovirus in any case of acute flaccid paralysis (AFP) was sufficient as proof of poliovirus in circulation – whether natural or introduced. Both are unwanted. Monitoring of eradication progress would have been much more straightforward and made much less expensive than the present situation in which all polioviruses in AFP cases have to be carefully analysed, and all polioviruses in sewage have to be detected and analysed. Sewage surveillance was necessitated only by polio occurrence due to VDPVs consequent to continued use of OPV, as we will explain below.

Wild polioviruses will show up, reasonably rapidly, as sudden onset paralysis of one or more limbs, – 'acute flaccid paralysis' (AFP) in other words; that is the reason for reliance on AFP surveillance as the monitoring method in polio eradication. VDPVs are less neurovirulent than wild polioviruses, and they may circulate widely before they may show up, causing AFP. We know that wild virus may cause one AFP for every 200-2000 infections. In other words, the case-to-infection ratio is 1/200 to 1/2000. Suppose high-quality AFP surveillance does not detect even one case during three years, in a whole country, with three annual birth cohorts free of polio. In that case, the likelihood of zero virus circulation is virtually cent per cent.

Vaccine viruses may probably cause one AFP (VAPP) for every 20,000-200,000 infections while VDPVs may cause one AFP for every 2000-20,000 infections. These numbers are guesstimates, but they illustrate why AFP surveillance is not sensitive enough to detect VDPVs through AFP surveillance alone. Sewage surveillance is essential.

If IPV was in use exclusively, poliovirus in any case of AFP had to be detected – without the need of sophisticated tests to distinguish wild from vaccine-like and vaccine-like from vaccine-derived. Any poliovirus, irrespective of its origin, would have been the signal of virus survival and movement in the community. There would have been no particular need for looking for polioviruses in sewage.

Vaccine and wild polioviruses -- friends and foes – wear the same uniform, so to say; they need to be identified and distinguished. That problem was created because of the blind belief in the faecal-oral transmission paradigm and the unproven assumption that OPV was essential to eradicate wild polioviruses. Thus, the basic question – nose or mouth – is not trivial but vital; if one is in the business of eradicating polio, the paradigm that explains all related phenomena is the right one. Faecal-oral does not, while respiratory does accommodate all related observations and phenomena.

Eradication strategy ought to have been wild-virus-centric

Eradication strategy ought to have been wild-virus-centric, not OPV-centric. Let us go back to 1988 when the decision was taken to eradicate polio globally. If the portal of entry were the nose, then IPV would have been the better choice, the ideal choice, especially in the longer term – we say longer-term only because OPV was already in widespread use at that time. OPV had to be ramped down, and IPV ramped up. The optimal time to replace all OPV with IPV was before 2000 or in 2000, the original target year for eradicating polioviruses --

irrespective of the prevalence of wild viruses somewhere and anywhere.

Creating polio in the name of curbing polio is irrational. It is also callous and cruel on the children and their families who need not have suffered life-long disability due to 'iatrogenic' (health-worker-caused) polio, while a perfectly safe alternative vaccine was already available and time tested. It is clearly contrary to public health ethics. In 1993 and thereafter in 1996 and during the 2000s, scientific publications indicated that OPV was not compatible with the very definition of polio eradication [3-5.]

All countries that eliminated all polio (wild virus and vaccine virus polio) had done so using IPV. So, attempting polio eradication using OPV exclusively is contrary to scientific evidence also. Once the year 2000 was missed, then the next earliest point in time to withdraw all OPV had to be considered and planned. Earlier would definitely have been better than later. Planning to continue OPV until after all wild viruses are globally eradicated had no 'all-weather safety' in it -- like putting a man on the moon and then thinking of how to bring him back. Many countries had eliminated wild virus polio using OPV but had to introduce IPV for withdrawing OPV. No country has eliminated wild viruses using OPV and then discontinued OPV without IPV in the system. Why take the world to the unknown, when an alternate safe strategy was already readily available?

That unscientific and unethical strategy design arose from the belief that creating intestinal mucosal immunity was the only way to eradicate wild polio viruses and OPV will be needed until the last transmission chain is stopped. That belief in the need for intestinal mucosal immunity arose from faith in the paradigm of faecal-oral transmission of wild polioviruses plus the fact that OPV is capable of inducing intestinal mucosal immunity. There is no scientific evidence that intestinal immunity is essential to stop wild poliovirus transmission. OPV is known to induce intestinal mucosal immunity; therefore, it was assumed that OPV should be relied upon to interrupt wild virus transmission - non sequitur. On the contrary, IPV was well known for its effectiveness to interrupt wild poliovirus transmission.

OPV is infectious – intestinal mucosal immunity is the body's response to any intestinal infection – typhoid fever, cholera, wild polioviruses or vaccine polioviruses. That does not mean a live vaccine is essential for individual protection, community control, regional elimination or global eradication. Observed facts did not support the essentiality for creating mucosal immunity by the live virus vaccine to interrupt wild virus transmission.

Evidence and belief were in contradiction. That is why we say that eradication should have been wild-virus-centric instead of OPV-centric. Once you choose OPV as essential, every attribute of OPV, such as intestinal mucosal immunity, is advertised as the reason for selecting OPV instead of IPV – simply, circular argument. Even the unwanted lateral spread of vaccine viruses was touted as an advantage of OPV over IPV; to call it advantage is oxymoron. Truly it was an unwanted disadvantage. Blind belief is a mental block to reckon with. If a vaccine virus spreads from the vaccinated to the unvaccinated, especially without their knowledge, the consequent infection has to be shown to be completely harmless. Laterally transmitted infection by vaccine poliovirus is not harmless.

Even if the portal of entry of wild poliovirus was thought to be the mouth (only for argument's sake), OPV would have been an acceptable choice only for the short term as it was already in use; it should not have been continued over longer-term, for reasons of the harmful biological properties of vaccine viruses. To answer the question of the route of transmission was, therefore, critical as the eradication strategy was being planned. The belief in oral route of infection was the reason for the perpetuation of OPV beyond its time limit. It was initiated on erroneous assumption. Well begun, the saying goes, is half done. Badly begun, or wrongly begun, is asking for trouble, delay, and over-demand of funds.

Reviewing the science and ethics of polio eradication

A review by the global polio eradication program to objectively examine the science and ethics of the strategy of polio eradication was wise as the interventions for eradication were being developed and applied in the field. There was such a review not by the program but by the International Epidemiological Association, held in Jerusalem in February 1993. One of the program organisers was Georgey Oblapenko, Medical Officer, Polio Eradication Unit of WHO Regional Office for Europe, Copenhagen, Denmark. The proceedings of that symposium were published in the international quarterly called Public Health Reviews, volume 21.[6] A proper review by the program itself, not other interested parties like the International Epidemiological Association, was due, nay, essential, latest by 2000, when the target year was reached without signs of early success. Such a review was designed and organised by, again, not the program, but by the Pasteur Institute in Paris – during 2000 June 28-30.[7] The Committee that planned its agenda included representatives of WHO and the Pan-American Health Organisation (PAHO, the WHO Regional Office for Americas). [7] Unfortunately, the visionary individual, Florian Horaud, who was the main force behind conceptualising the meeting, took ill and could not attend the meeting; he passed away on July 28, 2000.

The meeting did not function as consultation for strategy analysis and course correction planning, but merely as a scientific conference of many polio scientists. Experts from eradication program, from WHO and PAHO were very optimistic of the early success of eradication, and, in no mood to discuss the possibility of delay, failure, modification of strategy and tactics. Strong belief results in a closed mind or self-deception, leading to a denial of reality.

In the Paris meeting, the route of infection was argued to be nasal by one of us (TJJ), and the need and potential of IPV were clarified.[4,5] David Wood (rapporteur) stated: *"The global use of IPV for an interim period after global OPV cessation was strongly advocated by some discussants, but strongly opposed by others and remains the most controversial of the potential strategies"* [8]. The blind optimism of the program experts was clearly inappropriate for a public health program with so much at stake.

Note the words: *"global use of IPV...after global OPV cessation..."* The experts of the global polio eradication program did not get the message that IPV was necessary in order to stop OPV safely; hence it had to be in place before OPV cessation. The opinion of the majority of experts was that IPV had no role in global polio eradication.

Why has this 'most controversial' issue, a matter of 'life and death' for polio eradication, never been seriously analysed, debated, by the eradication program?

The premier global textbook on vaccines, "Vaccines," in its chapter on IPV in the 2008 edition, has the following statement: *"The role of IPV in facilitating eradication and its verification is much disputed, ranging from no role at all to complete substitution of IPV for OPV."*[9] No role for IPV was the opinion of polio eradication officials of the program. A complete substitution of OPV with IPV was the opinion of only one scientist [9].

Paradigm of faecal-oral transmission

The school of teaching on polio eradication that was guiding the program believed in the paradigm of faecal-oral transmission -- for oral entry of poliovirus there has to be a source that brings the virus to food and/or water. We know that polioviruses are shed in the throat secretions and in the stools of infected children. The argument for poliovirus reaching the mouth has to be the occurrence of faecal contamination of food or water. That paradigm had its beginnings with Sabin's teachings on the route and source of wild poliovirus transmission. Before Sabin's time, the general concept was that polioviruses were "highly contagious", "person-to-person transmitted" and, hence, inevitably respiratory transmitted, based on its worldwide distribution – someone had said 'democratic distribution'.

On the other hand, all microbes transmitted via a vehicle (non-respiratory route) such as food, water, insect bite and so on, are prevented by appropriate interventions to remove the vehicle or ensure that the vehicle does not get contaminated from the source of the microbe. It is precisely for this purpose, to prevent the entry of microbes from human and animal faeces, that sand filtration of drinking water was initiated in Britain and chlorination of drinking water in the USA during late nineteenth century or the early years of the twentieth century. All countries that supply safe potable water through piped distribution doing both – filtration plus chlorination, had eliminated almost all microbes transmitted by the faecal-oral route. But, as we said earlier, polio continued to occur and even caused outbreaks in all those countries until prevented, controlled and eliminated through immunization. Respiratory-transmitted infectious diseases are thus "exclusively vaccine-preventable"; that includes polio also.

Does the sun go around the earth, or does the earth go around the sun? Do wild polioviruses enter the body via the mouth or via the nostrils?

Flexner's studies on nasal entry of poliovirus.

Ask any polio expert as to who proved that wild polioviruses are transmitted via the faecal-oral route, and you will be answered that it was by Albert Sabin. That is what most people assume. Sabin did not prove that faecal-oral transmission was true or that respiratory transmission was not true. However, Sabin was able to convince most polio experts that wild poliovirus transmission was faecal-oral.

Not all polio experts were convinced, obviously. The Vellore school maintained nasal entry, the paradigm of the respiratory transmission, with the source being the wild viruses shed in the oral fluids of infected children as droplets and aerosol. Shedding of wild polioviruses in the throat is a consistent and undisputed fact. On the other hand, vaccine polioviruses colonise the upper respiratory tract poorly, and that may be a reason why they do not spread very efficiently.[10]

The devil was in the detail as we will explain below. If you think you know everything, you tend to overlook some detail. That is what actually happened. Scientists and leaders in high positions often think they know more than they actually know. Arrogance and biases then creep in and befuddle the interpretation of observations. *Observation is nothing; interpretation is everything.*

Scientists ought to be also 'prophets' of infectious diseases; both scientists and prophets observe the same things and both project into the future with the probabilities in mind. But true prophets are humble; scientists often are not. Unbiased interpretation requires an open mind and humility. Humility is always the best policy.

During the late nineteenth and early twentieth centuries, outbreaks of polio struck at unexpected places in Europe and the USA. In Vienna in 1908, Karl Landsteiner had proven that polio was caused by a 'virus'. Virus as we know it today had not been discovered, but virus was a name given by scientists with prophetic vision and precision. He had made an emulsion of the spinal cord of a child who had died of polio and filtered it through a porcelain filter that would retain all bacteria, and only 'virus' would pass through. Those days virus had not been visualised, as the electron microscope had not yet been invented. So virus was often qualified as 'filterable virus'. Landsteiner injected the emulsion into the stomachs of two Rhesus monkeys and both developed polio, and from their spinal cords, the filterable virus could be passed in fresh monkeys. Thus polio was proven to be a virus disease – the virus causing polio, when discovered, was given the name poliovirus.

Simon Flexner, famous for reforming medical education in the USA, was a pioneer polio researcher during the 1930s and 1940s. In 1932 he became the first Director of the Rockefeller Institute in New York. Simon Flexner was the first in the USA to repeat Landsteiner's method and collect poliovirus in the laboratory. But he inoculated the filtered spinal cord suspension of children who had died of polio, directly in the brains of monkeys. Then he passaged the virus serially in monkeys by brain inoculation. Viruses have a tendency to adapt to hosts and even host tissues when serially passaged. That phenomenon had a precedent: the experience of Louis Pasteur with the rabies virus.

He had serially passaged rabies virus in rabbits by the brain route, and the resultant strain was very different from the parent strain. Pasteur called the natural strain obtained from rabid dogs as "street virus" and the rabbit nervous tissue adapted one as "fixed virus". The latter was 'fixed' to the nervous system. Peripheral inoculation in the rabbit did not easily multiply, nor cause rabies, in rabbits or even dogs, unlike street virus. Pasteur had altered a basic property of the street rabies virus. He had attenuated rabies virus – thus was born the classical rabies vaccine.

Similarly, Flexner's poliovirus strain became infectious exclusively to the monkey's brain and spinal cord – it became a "fixed strain" to borrow the term from Pasteur. While Landsteiner could infect monkeys via the stomach, the virus in Flexner's laboratory, after many serial passages, would grow only in the brain or spinal cord -- strictly nervous tissue adapted, or exclusively 'neurotropic.'

During the 1930s and early 1940s, everyone had assumed that there was just one poliovirus – only much later, it was found that there were three poliovirus types, antigenically different from each other, numbered 1, 2, and 3.

What was the portal of entry of poliovirus in the monkey? Flexner found that he could infect monkeys and induce polio paralysis in them by swabbing the Rockefeller strain of poliovirus up the nasal canals of monkeys, but not by feeding them the virus orally.

He also found that the virus invaded the olfactory bulb, situated at the roof of the nasal cavity. The olfactory bulb has free-hanging nerve endings for the purpose of sensing smell. Poliovirus reached the brain via the olfactory bulb. So the route of entry of poliovirus in Nature was now 'established' as nasal, according to Simon Flexner. That concept fitted with the earlier epidemiological observations in many countries that poliovirus was highly contagious. But, there were a couple of twists in the tale.

What Flexner showed had three parts: one, the virus could infect monkeys via the nose. Second, the virus had to be swabbed into the nasal cavity, not inhaled as in real life. Third, then the virus reached the brain via the olfactory bulb and then from the brain to the spinal cord. All these were pertinent to the unique strain of the virus in hand – but that strain did not represent the "*street*" polioviruses in humans.

It was quite possible that poliovirus swabbing inoculated the olfactory bulb directly, without growing in nasal mucosal cells. Most contemporary virologists simply accepted Flexner's theory that poliovirus entered through the nose as it concurred with the known epidemiology of polio as it hit the rich and the poor. Polio was a big problem in the USA in spite of all care taken to sustain sanitation and hygiene.

Most children and adults who developed polio had no history of contact with another person with polio. That is easily explained as the vast majority of poliovirus infected persons are without the disease. But they act as a source of infection to others. Contact with silently infected persons is the most likely context of transmission. Poliovirus spreads stealthily. Respiratory transmission explained the likely sequence of events. We will illustrate this with the polio attack of Franklin D Roosevelt in 1921.

As a visionary leader, Flexner had hired very smart juniors including Albert Sabin, Thomas Francis Jr. and Tom Rivers. Only highly self-confident leaders would hire very smart juniors —less confident leaders tend to hire those who are unlikely to compete with themselves. Later on, in 1922, he hired Karl Landsteiner, who by then had become more interested in blood transfusion immunology and went on to describe the Rhesus blood group factor in the Rockefeller Institute. In 1930, as a member of the Rockefeller Institute, Landsteiner got the Nobel Prize for his discovery of blood groups and related factors that paved the way for safe blood transfusion as a life-saving medical intervention.

Sabin proved Flexner wrong

Albert Sabin, working in the Rockefeller Institute, had ready access to the stock of poliovirus, the Flexner's *"fixed"* (borrowing Pasteur's terminology) neurotropic strain. Sabin grew that strain in vitro in human embryonic brain tissue cultures, but it would not grow in non-neural tissues in culture. In those early days, to have poliovirus growing in any kind of tissue culture (even if exclusively brain tissue), was a convenience that avoided the need of expensive monkeys and chimpanzees for growing poliovirus.

The trio who actually showed that natural polioviruses grow in cell cultures (non-nervous tissue) from human foetuses were John Enders, Thomas Weller, and Frederick

Robbins. They were awarded the Nobel Prize for that breakthrough in 1954. Sabin had come so close to it, except that he did not know that the strain of poliovirus in Rockefeller Institute was an abnormal laboratory curiosity strain, not worth studying. Later in Jonas Salk's lab polioviruses were grown not only in human foetal skin cells, testicular cells, kidney cells – all non-neural tissue cells, but also in similar tissues from adult monkeys.

That the particular strain in Rockefeller Institute was not at all representative of poliovirus in Nature was not recognised by Sabin at that time or earlier by Flexner.

But Flexner's theory was not to Sabin's liking. According to Flexner's theory, a vaccine against polio would not work as poliovirus directly entered the nervous system via olfactory nerves.

In 1939 Sabin moved from New York to Cincinnati. He had shown poliovirus in plenty in the intestinal contents and in stools. He had proved that poliovirus infected the small intestine. He surmised (not with evidence) that the intestine was the initial (primary) site of poliovirus infection. He, therefore, interpreted the observations to mean poliovirus entered through the mouth. That made him convinced that a vaccine was realistic to protect against polio and that vaccine should be live attenuated orally fed vaccine.

But Flexner was the better-known scientist, and many had believed Flexner was right. Sabin began autopsy studies of children dying of polio – polio killed some 10% of affected children. All autopsy studies Sabin did, and he did dozens of them, showed no poliovirus in the olfactory bulbs. So Sabin demolished Flexner's theory. Sabin won the contest and was admired for his careful studies. David felled Goliath and was later chosen to be king by his people. Sabin defeated Flexner and became king in the world of polio research.

But there was a devil hiding in detail. What Sabin proved was only that polioviruses did not infect the olfactory bulb in children with polio. So, poliovirus could not have entered the nervous system via the olfactory bulb. That is all. In other words, what he actually proved was that in natural polio the olfactory bulb is not infected even though the strictly neurotropic poliovirus strain had infected the olfactory bulb in the monkey model -- no connection with the route of entry as nose or mouth. Flexner used nasal inoculation that resulted in olfactory bulb infection. Flexner's conclusion and Sabin's rebuttal were regarding the olfactory bulb as the route of virus entry from directly swabbed inoculation to the central nervous system. Nasal inoculation of that particular strain causing polio in monkeys has no bearing on the nasal transmission paradigm that we present.

Then there is the issue of the 'primary site' of infection. In every infectious disease, the microbe had to enter the human body (what epidemiologists call as inoculation and the route of inoculation) and initiate the process of infection at some anatomical site (called the site of primary infection). Route of inoculation and primary site of multiplication are basic in infectious disease epidemiology. Sabin interpreted intestinal infection to mean that site to be the primary site of infection and the route of inoculation to be, therefore, it's opening to the environment, namely the mouth. If intestines were the primary site of inoculation, oral entry is logical. But the primary site of multiplication is the pharynx. Intestines are the second or secondary site of infection and that inevitably results in shedding of poliovirus in the stools. Seeing poliovirus in the stool is not evidence that it entered by the mouth; non sequitur, we noted earlier

Where did Sabin go wrong?

Sabin's studies did not settle the question of the portal of entry. Sabin argued that the portal of entry was not the nose, for which he had no evidence. By now Sabin was the undisputed leader among all polio scientists. What he said had the ring of authority. We cannot judge if Sabin himself knew the flaw in his argument or not – but, he himself seemed to have been convinced of the oral entry of polioviruses. Most contemporary polio scientists swallowed Sabin's theory that the portal of entry of polioviruses was the mouth.

Polio epidemiologists have reason to believe that the primary site of infection is the pharynx – throat – which combines or crosses the respiratory pathway of air and alimentary pathway of food. Did Sabin look for poliovirus in throat secretions? Throat swab specimens are always positive for poliovirus in the infected child, but only for about two weeks in the early phase of infection. As soon as immunity develops throat shedding stops, but stool excretion continues for many more days to a few weeks in spite of immunity. That sounds odd, that infection and shedding continue for days and weeks in the face of immunity induced by pharyngeal infection.

Most people, including politicians, policymakers, Rotarians, philanthropists and most physicians, continue to believe in the faecal-oral paradigm of poliovirus transmission. *"Poliovirus enters the body through the mouth, travels down the digestive tract, and is excreted in the stools"* is a categorical statement in the book: Polio, An American Story.[10] That was the lesson taught by Sabin and learned by almost everyone else. *"Polio is an enteric (intestinal) infection, spread from person to person through contact with faecal waste: unwashed hands, shared objects, contaminated food, and water"*[11]

But in the same chapter in which the oral route is stated, there are some other statements that did not fit with faecal contamination of food or water as the risk factors of infection.

"Why did polio become epidemic in the twentieth century, a time when other infectious diseases were brought under control? And why did the most serious outbreaks occur in the advanced 'sanitary nations' of the West?"[11]

"Why was polio the most seasonal of afflictions, with thirty-five times as many cases in August as in April?"[11]

Regarding the investigation of Ivar Wickman in Stockholm, Sweden: *"Wickman was most interested in the transmission of the disease. With the skill of a medical detective, he traced the routes that carried the 'polio germ' from town to town along rural roads and railroad lines, and from child to child through contact at local schools. Polio was clearly contagious."* [11]Thiswas not influenza he was tracking, but Polio.

Regarding an outbreak of polio in Vermont in 1914: *"When examining key variables – nationality, prior diseases, population density, sewer facilities, water supply, condition of premises, domestic animals kept – health officials could find nothing to connect the victims beyond their age"*[11]

About an outbreak in New York City in 1916 with 8,900 cases and 2,400 deaths: *"In New York City, for example, public health officials found the epidemic to be most prevalent on Staten Island, which had the lowest population density and the best sanitary conditions of the city's five boroughs."*[11]

All the above descriptions fit perfectly for a respiratory-transmitted infection. However, the dogma remains that it is a faecal-oral infection.

Do not look for experimental proof

How would one prove that polioviruses entered via the nostril? To the best of our knowledge, no one has done either experiment – aerosol exposure of chimpanzees with wild poliovirus or of children with vaccine virus. Sabin had not proved that the natural portal of entry was the mouth, nor had he proved that the portal of entry was not the nose. But that was a convenient argument in favour of oral administration of live vaccine as if it mimicked Nature. Once Sabin disproved Flexner's theory, Sabin became the greatest polio expert, and most other polio scientists accepted his word.

Sabin was a brilliant scientist and a meticulous experimenter who hardly ever missed a detail. It is through meticulous observation of details and hard, patient and persistent laboratory work and animal inoculations that he ultimately developed the Sabin strains of attenuated polioviruses that became the OPV. Therefore, forgive us when we wonder if he himself truly believed in his teaching of oral virus entry or he had taught what he knew he had not proven. Did not Sabin eventually come to realise that the strain of poliovirus that infected the olfactory bulb turned out to be an odd, nervous-tissue-adapted, virus strain, non-representative of natural polioviruses and that all he proved was natural polioviruses did not invade the nervous system via olfactory bulb?

There was a 'glass wall' between brain invasion via olfactory bulb that Sabin disproved and the paradigm of respiratory transmission with nostrils as the portal of virus entry from droplets and aerosol of throat secretions/saliva of infected children that he did not investigate. Polioviruses infect the pharyngeal mucosa, and they are readily detected in infected children for about ten days to two weeks. Did Sabin know this or did he not? All polio experts know it.

In the 1960s in the USA, in the 1970s and 1980s in WHO polio committees and in all meetings – right until his demise he vehemently opposed any suggestion that his vaccine ever caused any polio – vaccine-associated paralytic polio (VAPP) -- in vaccinated, contacts or community-acquired. Did Sabin truly believe that Sabin viruses never caused VAPP, or was he simply and strongly defending his vaccine? We have not come across any other polio expert ever doubting that Sabin's vaccine indeed caused VAPP. By now he probably had assessed others – if they conflated uninfected olfactory bulbs with a non-nasal route of inoculation, just because of his authoritative word, he used the same tool to maintain that his vaccine was completely attenuated and totally safe.

Now we can see the probable source of the statement by even WHO, that OPV was one of the safest vaccines in use – statement from WHO committees with Sabin as a member.[12]

Window into Sabin's mind

Sabin very well knew that Sabin viruses were infectious from the vaccinated children to unvaccinated contacts. That did not always happen or even often, but it did happen occasionally. That presented a problem – actually two. In medical professionalism, you are not supposed to give a drug or vaccine to children without parental acceptance. Here was a vaccine that infected unsuspecting children who themselves were not being presented to be vaccinated.

What did Sabin do with that information? Very cleverly, he taught that such transmission was a good and desirable thing – more children than actually fed the vaccine will be immunised and protected. This was one of the dogmas Sabin propagated (as described in Chapter 5). So the decline in polio would be faster than what would account for vaccine coverage. That, Sabin taught, and others bought, would be a boon to developing countries in which the lateral spread would be more frequent than in developed countries on account of more chances of faecal-oral transmission. So you need not give OPV to 100% of children. Strange, that most experts actually believed that. The boon did not materialise; instead, it turned out bane. Even when, in most developing countries, the decline of polio burden was far slower than what was expected based on vaccine coverage, the experts maintained their belief, and, the evidence from observation was simply discarded. Even when such lateral spread was found to be the cause of polio in children, their faith remained unshaken. Such is the power of dogma and belief.

What is the reality? The decrease of polio in many developing countries was far less than what was expected for achieved vaccine coverage -- exactly the opposite of what Sabin taught. Also, there is less lateral spread in developing countries than in developed countries; actually, near-100% of children have to be fed OPV, again and again, to get most of them immune and protected.

The second problem was that the viruses in OPV that are fed by mouth and the viruses that came out in the stools were not the same in their neurovirulence characteristics. The viruses in stools were more neurovirulent than the vaccine viruses as Sabin himself had confirmed. Sabin also knew/ that even cell-culture passage in the laboratory tended to increase neurovirulence. So he had insisted that OPV should be made by using Sabin original viruses that had not been passed more than twice – SO+2 – Sabin original plus two cycles of cell culture amplification. To manufacture vaccine, one needs large amounts of seed virus to be grown in large laboratory ware. Sabin original as seed virus was not practical – it had to be amplified to make seed virus. SO+1 would not suffice; so SO+2. He knew that beyond SO+2 (or at most 3), OPV would have been 'hotter' – from neurovirulence viewpoint – not safe enough for non-immune children.

On the one hand, he denied VAPP as due to vaccine viruses, but yet he insisted on SO+2 for vaccine manufacture. If you refrain from questioning the authority, you have accepted the teaching as a dogma, and you blindly believe without need for evidence. Or, when evidence is inconvenient, vehemently defend the dogma.

The vaccine viruses in the vial were safer than those transmitted vaccine-progeny viruses from vaccinated children. Thankfully vaccine viruses do not transmit easily and for more than one or two generations. Still, it was better that all children were immunised with vaccine viruses from the vial than acquiring from other children. For that reason,

Sabin always recommended that OPV should be given in mass campaigns – so that the chances of vaccine virus transmission is minimised – all contact children would also have got the vaccine from vials.

All these are windows into Sabin's mind. Against this backdrop, will you blame us if we asked the question if Sabin was teaching the faecal-oral infection paradigm in spite of the fact that he only showed that the route of virus entry into the central nervous system was not the olfactory bulb? We understand why Sabin remained OPV-centric. Were his word and influence the reasons for polio eradication also becoming and remaining as OPV-centric?

Sabin had created the paradigm that that poliovirus entered through the mouth and grew in the intestines. Growing in the intestine was true and objectively proved. As for entering through the mouth we are sure of only vaccine viruses that enter through the mouth. They are fed by mouth. There is no direct evidence that the route of entry of wild polioviruses is the mouth. There is also no indirect evidence. It remains a dogma. We must learn to distinguish between dogma and evidence-based conclusion.

Spurious arguments to support the faecal-oral paradigm

The believers of the faecal-oral paradigm supported their belief by yet another unproven assumption, that there was more polio in communities with poor hygiene and sub-standard sanitation than in countries with good sanitation and hygiene, because of the greater likelihood of faecal-oral transmission. That was one of the supportive arguments for faecal-oral paradigm. The observation was partially true – only partially true, but not for the attributed reason.

In the pre-vaccine era, there was an observation that polio was less common in countries with poor sanitation and hygiene than in developed and cleaner countries. That was also partially true – if you counted cases and ignored poliovirus infections. When infants got infected while maternal antibody was still present in the infant's blood, infants were protected against polio paralysis in spite of infection. But that infection-induced infant's own antibody response that was long-lasting. Such children did not develop polio later on. In developing countries, the speed of spread of wild polioviruses was faster than in developed countries. That resulted in early infections and overall less disease.

So, what differed between some developing countries and some developed countries was the speed of spread of wild polioviruses. And, the speed of spread was determined by the density of the childhood population, which in turn is determined by both population density and birth rate.

The observed fact of less polio in developing countries during the pre-vaccine era was true but illusory if extrapolated to infections; there were no fewer poliovirus infections than in rich countries. As a respiratory-transmitted infection, everyone got infected in high-population-density developing countries. In developed countries the speed of transmission was slower; hence cases were apparently more and at higher ages. In developing countries, polio was compressed essentially between five months and five years of age. Infection below five months would not cause polio because of protection from the maternal antibody. In developed countries, young children, older children, adolescents and even adults developed polio because of the slow spread of infection. The total number of cases per unit population, what statisticians call the denominator, was not very different. In Finland and the USA (before vaccination controlled polio) and in India, about 20 cases per 100,000 population per year was the observed numbers. That meant that 1 in 1000 per year had polio – in developing countries all concentrated in the under-five age group but in developed countries spread over 30-40 years of life.

In some developed countries, there was less polio per unit population partly because some had totally escaped poliovirus infection due to the slow spread. Due to slow spread, not the entire population was saturated by infection. When adults developed polio we knew that the speed of infection was indeed slow. In developing countries, on the other hand, infection and the cases of polio saturated the children by age five years. Hardly anyone developed polio beyond five years of age.

The birth rate is another factor – another devil of a detail. The higher the birth rate, the more susceptible heads per unit population, added each year. That meant more polio per unit population taken in toto. The lower the birth rate, the less is the proportion of the susceptible population – that meant less polio. Remember, polio was ubiquitous and not geographically restricted to communities with a lack of safe drinking water or safe disposal of excreta.

In the eradication era, the assumption was turned on its head to depict more polio attributed to poor hygiene that goes parallel to the faecal-oral transmission of many other infections, particularly those that cause diarrhoea. Indeed there was more polio, but the reason was not faecal-oral transmission, but polio had been controlled with vaccines in hygienic countries which had robust immunization programmes as well.

Why should a respiratory transmitted infection differ in speed between different countries? During the 1930s, 1940s, and 1950s, there were polio outbreaks in many rich countries with good hygiene, safe disposal of excreta and provision of safe drinking water. From less polio the epidemiology changed to more polio, especially periodically as outbreaks. Then the explanation was that good hygiene had earlier slowed down the speed of spread; consequently, older children eventually got infected, and there is a tendency for more disease per number of infections in the older children, adolescents and young adults. This was the 'hygiene hypothesis' or 'development hypothesis' of the new phenomenon of polio outbreaks in the 20th century in rich countries. Developing countries did not have any appreciable change in their steady-state of polio epidemiology.

All such shifting sand assumptions did not take into account the confounding factor that differing birth rates and densities of population determined the differences in polio epidemiology in different countries. The more crowded, and the higher the birth rate, the more the density of child population. Infections transmitted via the respiratory route tend to move faster in such populations.

Has anyone looked at birth rates or population densities as determinants of the distribution of cases by numbers and by age? Yes, indeed, a few have.

Influence of birth rates and population densities on poliovirus transmission

In North America and in Europe, many countries faced outbreaks of polio during the first half of the twentieth century, as a new phenomenon without explanation. Most experts suspected that the 'age shift' of polio, with infants escaping polio and getting exposed as grown-ups, was the paradoxical effect of good hygiene. That was the 'hygiene hypothesis' or 'development hypothesis'.

One astute observer had identified the post-world war 'baby boom' as the main reason for the changing epidemiology and disease burdens. With low numbers of babies to amplify polioviruses, not everyone got infected with polioviruses, especially as living conditions were good. With the baby boom, the epidemiology of infection changed – infants and young children amplified the viruses and pretty much everyone was exposed. The more the infection burden, the more the disease burden.

The person who showed the connection between the baby boom and shifting polio epidemiology was Jane S Smith. She was neither a scientist nor a polio expert. She wrote the book "Patenting the Sun: Polio and the Salk vaccine."[13]

We quote from her book: *"In the decade from 1945 to 1955, the years that saw most of the research that made the Salk vaccine possible, two unrelated movements came together to magnify the importance of the National Foundation [for Infantile Paralysis]. The first was a steady, visible rise in the number of cases of polio. The second was the postwar population explosion commonly known as the Baby Boom."*[13]

She then gave the numbers of births in the Baby Boom years to support her viewpoint in the book. We quote again: *"To the biostatisticians who kept track of these figures, the parallel rise of birth rate and epidemic rate [of polio] was an insignificant coincidence. Coincidence it may have been, but it was hardly insignificant."*[13]

Most polio experts had missed the connection between population densities, birth rates, and polio rates -- then and during the eradication era as well. The moment you accept the connection, the elephant stands out – transmission has got to be respiratory. How easy it was, and is, to miss the elephant in the room!

Many decades later, an elegant study by Martinez-Bakkar, King and Rohani, published in 2015, has corroborated Jane Smith's conclusion. The title of the publication was: "Unravelling the transmission ecology of polio"[14]. We quote from the abstract: *"Contrary to the prevailing 'disease of development hypothesis' our analyses demonstrate that polio's historical expansion was straightforwardly explained by demographic trends rather than improvements in sanitation and hygiene."*

The hypothesis that the increase in polio in western countries was due to improved sanitation and hygiene – the 'disease of development' hypothesis – was based on the paradigm of faecal-oral transmission. That paradigm is full of anomalies.

We once again quote from the Authors' summary: *"Historical epidemics that predate the use of vaccines can be used to disentangle the epidemiology of disease from vaccine effects. Using historical polio data from large-scale epidemics in the US, we fitted and simulated mathematical models to track poliovirus and reconstruct the millions of unobserved subclinical infections that propagated the disease. We identified why polio epidemics are explosive and seasonal and why they vary geographically. Our analyses show that the historical expansion of polio is straightforwardly explained by the demographic 'baby boom' during the post-war period rather than improvements in hygiene."*[14]

The Pasteur Institute in Paris had hosted the international symposium titled, "Progress in Polio Eradication: Vaccine Strategies for the End Game", during 28-30 June 2000, as mentioned earlier. In that symposium, Isao Arita of smallpox eradication fame argued that population density was a critical factor in the ease or difficulty of interruption of transmission of both smallpox and polio[15]. We quote: *"Low density of population...may explain why some national programmes have rapidly stopped polio transmission by rather mediocre immunization program and surveillance. The best examples have been in Bolivia, Papua New Guinea and Southern African Countries. The density of population in most of these countries is extremely low, being less than 10-30 per [sq] km. Likewise, many countries in sub-Saharan Africa have a low population density. Thus, sub-Saharan Africa may enjoy a guarded optimism for stopping polio transmission by 2002. Sometimes transmission may die out naturally [where population density is very low]. However, there are some circumstances, which might cause a delay. For example, the density of population in Nigeria is 125 per [sq] km, the highest in sub-Saharan Africa. As of May 2000, the disease was highly endemic there. In smallpox eradication, Nigeria was also the last endemic country in entire West Africa despite its better health system"* [15, pages:37-38]

Arita's observation was astute, accurate, and interpretation impeccable. His conclusions do have a ring of authenticity, authority. His interpretation was 'prophetic'. People and prophets see the same things, but prophets perceive more than people. Nigeria is the one country in all of Africa that has resisted every attempt to evict wild polioviruses until 2012 (type 3) and 2016 (type 1).

Arita had also pointed out that *"in all India, the three northern states with the highest density [of] population, Uttar Pradesh, Bihar and West Bengal were or have been resistant to the eradication efforts both in smallpox and polio".*

The very last cases of smallpox and of polio in India were in these very same states. If population density, especially the density of population of infants and under-five children, is a determinant of the tenacity of the target virus, or the ease of its interruption, the route of its transmission cannot be faecal-oral, but respiratory: as for smallpox, so for polio too.

The position of WHO experts of the Western School

The WHO position papers on polio vaccines consistently state that polioviruses are transmitted via the faecal-oral pathway (polio vaccine position papers of 2014 and 2016)[16,17]. In recent years 'oral-oral' transmission pathway is also added in the position papers.[16,17]

Entry by mouth is a tenet of belief in polio epidemiology among all OPV believers. The oral-oral pathway is a silly proposition – children with poliovirus infection do not go around kissing other children to transmit poliovirus.

Epstein-Barr virus and meningococcal bacteria may be present in the throats of adolescents, and by kissing these two agents may readily get transmitted. They are oral-oral transmitted. As for polioviruses, the oral-oral transmission is a far-fetched and an unrealistic proposition.

The oral-oral theory became necessary because there is the presence of poliovirus in the oral fluids of all infected children – when a microbe is shed into the environment a particular way, there is usually a consequence to that mode of shedding. All epidemiologists recognise that. So, combine oral virus and Sabin-dogma of oral entry – oral-oral is the inevitable conclusion even if that is like the spider and flies story. Everything is not what it seems to be.

The scary side of the story is that no one else seems to be concerned about such a weird proposition. That suggests absolute faith in the experts and their assertions – on the part of most people involved in polio eradication.

We are aware of one instance of oral-oral transmission of polio. Dr Gwenda Lewis was head of anaesthesia department in Christian Medical College from 1947. When there was a child in respiratory distress, in October 1953, she gave mouth-to-mouth breathing to revive the child – and within a few days, she got polio paralysis of both legs. Such oral-oral spread might have happened very occasionally – but children getting polio due to oral-oral spread is most unlikely, to say the least.

Paradigm of respiratory transmission

Let us explain our concept of nasal transmission of poliovirus. All textbooks state that wild polioviruses are highly contagious – meaning easily transmitted 'person to person'. That actually implies that it is not transmitted by faecal contamination of food or water.

In countries with high population density and high birth rate, children develop poliovirus infection very early in life. By age five they are saturated with the first (and immunising) infection with all three polioviruses.[18]

Imagine polioviruses in droplets of oral fluids or aerosol. A few virus particles are inhaled. Being some 20-25 nanometers in size, they go past the nostrils and enter deep inside. It would take just one poliovirus to touch the surface of a cell that is susceptible to infection – bingo; the child is infected. One infected cell releases more than 10,000 virus particles. Other neighbouring cells get infected, and the process continues. Every time the child swallows, polioviruses are also swallowed. Then the intestinal mucosa gets infected – probably, we guess, after umpteen times when the virus could not infect the intestines. Then one time the intestine gets infected.

This concept will explain how children in India (and Pakistan, Nigeria) are easy targets for wild polioviruses even when they fail to get infected when a million vaccine poliovirus particles are fed by mouth in OPV drops. Direct oral inoculation of vaccine polioviruses is not very efficient in establishing infection in many low-income countries. If the nose was the portal of entry of wild poliovirus, and if pharynx got infected first, then the intestinal infection would automatically follow.

In this way, we consider the pharynx as the 'primary site of infection', and site of early virus multiplication, soon followed by intestinal infection and copious amounts of poliovirus shed in the stools. Thus intestine is the 'secondary site' of multiplication, not the primary. If that is so, oral entry (for primary infection in intestines) is not relevant; nasal entry will result in intestinal infection in a short while.

Upper respiratory symptoms of poliovirus infection

What are the early symptoms of wild poliovirus infection in children? This question cannot be easily answered unless careful observations and virological investigations are made in clinical settings and situations. The USA is one country that had collected such information over many years; the detailed clinical description was essential for research on polio in the pre-vaccine era.

Experts categorised the clinical effect of poliovirus infection at the USA Centers for Disease Control and Prevention – CDC Atlanta, as (1) inapparent or asymptomatic; (2) minor, nonspecific illness; (3) non-paralytic aseptic meningitis; and (4) paralytic polio. These are arranged in the decreasing order of frequency[17]. We quote: *"Approximately 4%-8% of polio infections consist of a minor, nonspecific illness without clinical or laboratory evidence of central nervous system invasion. This clinical presentation is known as abortive poliomyelitis and is characterised by complete recovery in less than a week. Three syndromes observed with this form of poliovirus infection are*

- *upper respiratory tract infection (sore throat and fever),*
- *gastrointestinal disturbances (nausea, vomiting, abdominal pain, constipation or, rarely diarrhoea), and*
- *influenza-like illness.*

These syndromes are indistinguishable from other viral illnesses."[19]

The fact that poliovirus infection may cause symptoms of an upper respiratory tract infection and of influenza is suggestive and supportive of the concept of respiratory transmission rather than faecal-oral transmission.

Many other enteroviruses cause human infections. Among all enteroviruses some are inactivated by acidity in the stomach, while others are not. Those that are acid-labile do not survive the acidity in the stomach – and do not infect the intestinal tract. They do not get excreted in the stool – Enterovirus D68 is a good example. It is respiratory transmitted – via droplets or aerosol of oral/nasal fluids. It is acid-labile and not found in stool.

Some enteroviruses (Coxsackie A 16 and Enterovirus 71, for example) that cause a syndrome – hand foot and mouth syndrome – are notoriously highly contagious, via respiratory tract (inhaled aerosol/droplets). All of them are also shed much in stools. Many enteroviruses (Coxsackievirus, echovirus serotypes) are well known to cause upper respiratory tract illness resembling common cold and sore throat.

It is most unlikely that there are any enteroviruses that are exclusively faecal-oral transmitted. All enteroviruses, well, almost all, are ubiquitous, present and endemic in all countries. All ubiquitous viruses are respiratory transmitted – otherwise, they would be geographically restricted and die out in hygienic populations of rich countries.

How did Roosevelt catch polio?

The front-page story in New York Times on September 16, 1921, was: "F. D. Roosewelt Ill of Poliomyelitis; Brought on Special Railroad Car from Campobello, Bay of Fundy, to Hospital Here. Recovering, Doctors say."[11]

Franklin D Roosevelt, during the 1921 polio season, in summer, attended a youth group in New York – a Boys Scout celebration in Hyde Park, New York.[11] He addressed them and mingled with them. A few days later, Roosevelt developed bilateral lower limb paralysis that was typical of polio, with muscle aches and very rapid progression.

Polio was indeed contagious – except that more than 99% of infected persons remain well, but only an occasional person became paralysed. Polioviruses had not been discovered in 1921. Some child was infected and passed on that infection to Roosevelt. Respiratory transmission was most likely. We must point out that some have questioned if Roosevelt's illness was polio. All available clinical details, particularly the severe muscle aches, were typical of polio and not typical of the suggested alternate diagnosis of Guillain-Barre syndrome.

Fact is that infected children shed wild polioviruses both in oral fluids that are expelled as droplets and aerosol, as well as in stools. So, the virus in the air could be inhaled. But what are the chances of the virus in stools actually reaching the mouths of children? Which of the two was the normal source of infection in new hosts?

If the eradication program was designed well, theoretically, actually either vaccine would have been effective in interrupting wild virus transmission, with a caveat. In countries where the vaccine efficacy of OPV was very low, using OPV to interrupt transmission of wild polioviruses would have been predictably an uphill task. Uphill, like what Sisyphus was cursed to do – roll up a stone to the top and as its rolls back down, repeat the task again and again. The same children had to be contacted and fed OPV, again and again, many times – 10-40 times. In such countries, IPV was the better choice irrespective of the route of transmission, as it would have been sufficient to vaccinate children just three times. Then why was OPV used exclusively? Those who go by faith tend to over-defend their position. We have no other explanation. As in religion, so also in science, faith can overrule evidence by the followers.

The lesson that the task of interrupting wild virus transmission using OPV was uphill was learned the hard way – in countries like India, Egypt, Niger, Nigeria, Democratic Republic of Congo, Sudan, Ethiopia, Afghanistan and Pakistan. The reason why the eradication program insisted and persisted using only OPV was for the reason of the belief in the faecal-oral transmission paradigm. As the route of transmission was not faecal-oral but respiratory -- the entire struggle with continued use of only OPV was unnecessary.

The route of entry of natural polioviruses made a world of difference for the eradication program. The faecal-oral transmission paradigm was illusory -- there was no scientific evidence for the validity of the paradigm. All circumstantial evidence was overwhelmingly in favour of respiratory transmission paradigm.

The slippery slope of faecal-oral transmission paradigm

Those who believed in the faecal-oral transmission paradigm made one more assumption that was purely theoretical. That assumption was most probably the reason why the global polio eradication program chose to use OPV exclusively for local polio elimination in developing countries and global polio eradication. The assumption was that creating 'intestinal immunity' was a necessary step in interrupting wild poliovirus transmission.

Like the paradigm itself, this assumption also had no scientific basis. Intestinal infection with wild or vaccine viruses induces intestinal immunity. All intestinal infections induce intestinal immunity against their respective microbes. However, intestinal immunity in most infections, including wild poliovirus infections and vaccine poliovirus infections, is not only incomplete or partial but also relatively short-lived. Most such infections may occur again when exposed, especially after intestinal immunity has waned. This is true even for polioviruses.

Intestinal immunity definitely reduces the quantum and duration of wild virus shedding in the stool when 'challenged' again – with wild viruses or vaccine viruses. That is a normal phenomenon. However, there is no evidence – laboratory or community – that intestinal immunity is essential, at least necessary, or even helpful, in interrupting the chains of transmission of wild polioviruses. The fact that some countries were able to interrupt wild virus transmission with only IPV, was evidence contrary to the assumption that intestinal immunity was necessary to control and eliminate polio. The evidence was mentally suppressed to avoid cognitive dissonance, so to say, and the belief in the faecal-oral paradigm was kept up with greater vigour than before.

To repeat: the assumption that intestinal immunity is necessary for interrupting wild poliovirus transmission was the rationale of the exclusive use of OPV in the eradication strategy, with all its many problems that have come to haunt the program over the years. There was no evidence that intestinal immunity was important for interrupting wild virus transmission. The country models of elimination in Europe had already proved that IPV was sufficient, indeed efficient, to interrupt wild virus transmission and to eliminate polio.

For those who believed in the respiratory transmission paradigm, creating intestinal immunity was unnecessary, unimportant – actually a misleading distraction. It did not matter very much how much wild virus was shed in the stools of children, as virus in faeces does not necessarily enter the food and water consumed by children everywhere.

Polio, like measles, is an exclusively vaccine-preventable disease. No amount of environmental sanitation, efficient sewage system for safe disposal of human excreta, quality assured safe drinking water without any faecal contamination – none of these could prevent polio, even polio in outbreaks. Polio continued to occur where all other faecal-oral pathogens were prevented and controlled to the point of elimination. Polio was not a disease only of countries with poor sanitation. Polio was ubiquitous until vaccines were used against it.

We say that in most situations faeces is not the actual source of virus for transmission, although if faecal contamination of food or water was heavy, the transmission is possible. No one has proved that – we can only guess. That is an experiment that cannot be done.

OPV infects when given by the mouth; therefore, the wild virus also may infect if given by mouth. However, you cannot feed the wild virus, but you can give OPV to a child already given OPV and shown to have been immune. What do you think happens? In many if not most instances, the child gets infected once again. So, immunity induced by OPV is not absolutely protective against a subsequent infection, even with vaccine viruses. However, the quantum of the virus in the stools would be far less than what is found after the first feeding when the child was not immune. Also, the duration of shedding is cut down to a much shorter duration. That is the result of intestinal immunity.

Those who believed in the paradigm of faecal-oral transmission used this argument to support their assumption that intestinal immunity was absolutely essential for interrupting wild virus transmission. What would happen if the OPV-protected children are exposed to wild polioviruses? Although that cannot be tested, there have been several 'natural experiments' in communities that were well-vaccinated and polio very much controlled.

Effect of importation of poliovirus in well-vaccinated community

When wild poliovirus is re-introduced and begins spreading, children, themselves immune from paralytic polio, have acted as links in chains of transmission of wild polioviruses resulting in polio outbreaks in well vaccinated (with OPV or IPV) countries. The interesting difference is that such introduction causes no polio in IPV immunised countries/communities but sporadic and even outbreak polio is common in OPV immunised countries/communities.

We quote Peter Patriarca[20] *'The first of these outbreaks was reported from Taiwan in 1982 where 1031 poliomyelitis cases (5.8 cases per 100,000 total population) were identified over a 6-month period.21 Although 65% of these cases occurred in unvaccinated infants, estimates of the rate of infection suggested that children who had received three or more doses of OPV, although protected from paralysis, none the less participated in the chain of transmission.22*

Similar findings were subsequently reported following investigations of type 1 outbreaks in The Gambia in 198623 and Oman in 1988-89.24 Indeed laboratory-based investigations following a cluster of type 1 cases in Cartagena, Columbia in

1990 found similar rates of asymptomatic poliovirus infection in both fully vaccinated and unvaccinated infants (JK Andrus et al. unpublished data) ".

So intestinal immunity is a phenomenon, all right, but it does not seem to be a very relevant phenomenon for interrupting wild virus circulation. Taiwan and The Gambia reports were available before the World Health Assembly resolution in 1988. The Oman and Columbia data were available to the eradication program experts before 2000.

We know very little about the biologic and epidemiological function of intestinal immunity. Children given OPV respond with immune responses by the second week. The peak immunity is by the third week. However, such children may keep on shedding vaccine viruses in the stool for four weeks, in some cases 6 weeks, and in other cases up to 8 or even ten weeks. So children keep on excreting the virus in the face of strong intestinal immunity, no one knows why.

However, virus shedding in the throat ceases as soon as immunity develops. By day ten, after the onset of polio in a child, the throat is clear of virus, but virus shedding in the stool continues for another 2-10 weeks. This is suggestive, but not proof, that Nature has endowed immunity sufficient to prevent further transmission – as throat shedding ceases.

IPV induces better pharyngeal protection than OPV and is more efficient in interrupting wild virus transmission. IPV had other advantages also – like (1) very limited number of doses being sufficient for long-lasting immunity; (2) Expanded Program on Immunization (EPI) could have been used as IPV delivery platform; (3) complete safety from serious adverse events following immunization.

If IPV through EPI was the backbone of the eradication strategy, OPV could have been used at will, as needed, where needed, and then withdrawn for avoiding the continued seeding of the community with polioviruses – eradication was to remove polioviruses from the community.[25]

One well known and well-studied episode of re-introduction of WPV into an IPV-using country is what happened in Israel in 2013.[26] The country had been on exclusive IPV use since 2005. As sewage was regularly sampled and tested for various microbes, WPV type 1 was detected to be circulating silently in the country – from 2013 February till 2014 April. Its source was most probably Nigeria. Israel conducted nation-wide monovalent type 1 OPV campaign targeting all children below 10, with two doses two months apart. Epidemiological analysis suggested that the OPV campaign interrupted virus transmission. Two important lessons are that there was not even a single case of polio in the population, illustrating the exquisite vaccine efficacy of IPV against polio disease and that OPV campaigns are feasible to interrupt WPV transmission if WPV is re-introduced.

It was only because of sewage surveillance the WPV infection outbreak was detected. If such episodes had happened in other IPV-using countries without sewage surveillance, no one would know.

Finland is a country that uses only IPV and has also sewage surveillance. In 2013, vaccine-derived poliovirus types 1 and 2 were detected several times.[27] These outbreaks of infection were silent, without causing any polio. The viruses were genetically related to earlier sewage isoltes during 2008-2012. Sewage in Israel also had shown the presence of VDPV 1 and 2 occasionally. The true sources of these VDPVs have not beel pinpointed.

Importance of respiratory transmission to the eradication program

If the respiratory transmission was natural and common, OPV was not important, but if it had to be used, it should have been used only for a very short term, not longer than absolutely necessary. As the target date was 2000, the strategy should have been that OPV was discontinued before or by 2000 or shortly thereafter.

Both wild viruses and vaccine viruses are the cause of polio. Beyond 2000 vaccine viruses should not have been allowed to cause any polio as 2000 was the target date set for polio eradication. Continuing to give a polio-inducing virus beyond the target date was against the spirit of the 1988 WHA resolution that had set the time target of the year 2000.

Had the Western school accepted the respiratory transmission paradigm, or at least considered it worthy of consideration as a probable or at least possible paradigm, the entire polio eradication strategy would have been drastically different.

Then there would not have been the obsession to create intestinal mucosal immunity for which OPV was promoted for exclusive use. The belief in the faecal-oral transmission paradigm led to the exclusive use of OPV that has resulted in most of the problems facing the eradication program before 2000, since 2000, even today in 2020. That assumption has resulted in inequity – rich countries using IPV and poor countries using OPV and suffering from vaccine-induced polio – both sporadic and outbreak.

Which paradigm is more probable?

There is no direct or experimental evidence for either paradigm. It would be unethical to inoculate anyone with wild polioviruses by the nose or by the mouth. Therefore we have to rely on circumstantial observations and pieces of evidence.

The major argument in favour of oral route of entry is that vaccine polioviruses in OPV infect children when given by mouth. All polioviruses, wild, vaccine and vaccine-derived, belong to one species. If vaccine viruses infect by mouth, it is reasonable to assume that wild viruses also could infect by mouth. However, our question is not if wild viruses could infect by mouth but do they actually infect by mouth under natural conditions. Several pieces of information suggest that wild viruses do not ordinarily get in through the mouth, as we have elaborated above.

A dose of trivalent OPV contained at least one million infectious particles of type 1 Sabin strain, at least 100,000 infectious particles of type 2 Sabin strain and at least 600,000 infectious particles of type 3 Sabin strain. Even with such high virus content, in India, only some 10-30% of children got infected with type 1 and type 3 Sabin viruses after consuming a dose of OPV. In order to immunise near-100% children with types 1 and 3 vaccine viruses, some 10 to 30 doses were required. At the same time, children in India were highly susceptible to wild virus infection even at such a young age as early infancy. Fifty per cent of children were infected with all three types of wild viruses by 12-15 months of age.

A child shedding wild poliovirus in stools would have about 1000 to 10,000 live virus particles in a gram of faeces. Let us assume that if tested at the right time after infection, there could be a time when 100,000 live virus particles may be shed per gram of stool. In order to get 100,000 to a million wild virus particles going into the mouth of an infant, one to 10 grams of faeces need to be ingested. Even one gram of stool contaminating a child's feed is simply an absurd possibility; it is simply impossible.

Moreover, most infants are breastfed until about six months of age. Then weaning food – always cooked food except for fruits – is given in very small amounts and gradually increased in quantity. Infancy, therefore, is the least likely age when food or water heavily contaminated with faeces will get into the baby. The fastest increase in the frequency of wild poliovirus infection used to be between 6 and 12 months when the likelihood of faecal contamination of weaning food is extremely low. It is, therefore, most unlikely, if not impossible, that faecal-oral route is applicable for polioviruses in the very young, the usual age of wild poliovirus infection in children in countries like India.

If a very high dose of Sabin virus does not infect our children readily, then common sense tells us that our children should have been less prone to infection with the wild virus too. They are variants of the same species. If that were true, we would have had less polio, overall, in young children than in countries in which the infection frequency of vaccine viruses was much higher. The opposite was true: we had a higher incidence of polio in young children than in countries with a better immune response to Sabin viruses. So, we have a dichotomous or a paradoxical situation – high infection susceptibility with wild polioviruses and low infection susceptibility with vaccine polioviruses. This does not make sense unless the routes of entry of the two are different – oral for vaccine viruses but nasal for wild viruses.

Before polio vaccination was widely applied, polio in children began to appear in India from about five months of age (after the decline of maternal antibody), and 50% of children who had polio had it by 12-15 or maximum 18 months of age -- called 'median age' of polio. By age five years, the risk of polio was virtually over – that meant that virtually 100% of children had been infected with wild polioviruses types 1, 2 and 3. So, wild virus found children very easy targets, while we found it difficult to infect children with Sabin poliovirus – this paradox told us to be cautious about concluding that oral route as the natural route of entry of wild poliovirus.

Interestingly, the above age pattern of infection is nearly identical to that of measles before the time the measles vaccine became widely used. Measles is undoubtedly a respiratory transmitted infection. Maternal antibody against measles survives in the infant a bit longer than is the case for maternal antibody against polioviruses. So, cases of measles begin to show up from 5-6 months of age and the median age of measles used to be about two years, even higher than that of polio. The speed with which polioviruses infected infants was faster than the speed with which measles virus infected children in India. Polio was more contagious than measles. This transmission dynamics could not have been created by faecal-oral transmission. It stands to reason that polioviruses are respiratory transmitted viruses.

Faecal-oral transmission is determined by the chances and 'doses' of faecal contamination of drinking water or food. And we do have many instances of such contamination in various communities at various times. But we do not have faecal contamination in every community and at all times. Polioviruses saturate children in most if not all developing countries with infection by age five years, no matter rich or poor, urban or rural. Such saturation, virtually 100 % of children getting infected, can occur only with the respiratory transmission. So, the simplistic argument that vaccine viruses infect after swallowing OPV is not proof enough that stool contamination in food or water, in other words, faecal-oral route, is the way infants got infected with wild polioviruses.

The virus content in OPV is in grossly unnatural quantities, not in natural quantities that infants and children get exposed to in Nature. In the case of other live virus vaccines, measles, rubella, and mumps – 1000 virus particles are sufficient to infect and immunise most children – but these are always injected.

Finding plenty of polioviruses in stools of children does not mean that faecal-oral has to be the route of transmission. Polioviruses are also shed in throat and saliva; how could we believe that such shedding is irrelevant for the spread of polioviruses?

There are microbes well known to be transmitted by the faecal-oral route. Bacteria causing typhoid fever, cholera, dysentery; and viruses causing acute hepatitis A and E are classic examples of microbes that are shed in the stool but not in nasal or pharyngeal secretions. Only if faeces contaminate food or water can such infections spread. Where sanitation and hygiene are excellent, such infections do not occur as they would have died out for want of channels of transmission. Where sanitation and hygiene are poor, faecal-oral infections and diseases due to them are frequent.

All known microbes with faecal-oral transmission cause food-borne and water-borne outbreaks whenever there was a breach in sanitation, water-safety or food hygiene. We have never heard of a food-borne or water-borne outbreak of polio anytime, anywhere. Even when drinking water is heavily contaminated with faces, as evidenced by outbreaks of such diseases – hepatitis A, hepatitis E, typhoid fever, cholera – polio outbreak has never occurred during such times.

Countries that became rich before or during the early 20th century established safe disposal of human excreta and supply of safe drinking water. Examples are many European and the two North American countries. They all once had common diseases caused by faecal-oral microbes – cholera, typhoid fever, dysenteries, hepatitis A etc. All of these virtually disappeared with the 'great sanitary movement' that began in the 19th century in European and North American countries. On the other hand, polio did not. Polio remained ubiquitous and caused outbreaks in all countries during the 20th century.

Scandinavian countries such as Finland, Norway, Sweden and Iceland are the best examples of countries with near-perfect sanitation and hygiene; yet, during early and mid-20th century all of them had a high incidence of polio, with even large outbreaks in some years. The same was true in the USA and Canada. The urgency for developing a vaccine to protect from polio was precisely that. IPV was available from 1955 onwards. Once Scandinavian countries began using IPV, they were able to eliminate polio due to wild polioviruses. For such epidemiological reasons, polio had earned the qualification as an 'exclusively vaccine-preventable' disease.

Improvements in sanitation and hygiene did not affect polio prevalence.

All other 'exclusively vaccine-preventable' diseases are respiratory transmitted – measles, mumps, rubella, chickenpox, smallpox, influenza, pneumonia caused by *pneumococcus* and *Haemophilus influenza* b etc. And vaccines have been created against all of them. There are others without a vaccine, but we do not enumerate them here.

Another fascinating point: vaccines against *pneumococcus* and *Haemophilus influenzae* type b – and also against whooping cough and diphtheria, exhibit a remarkable degree of 'herd effect'. Herd effect is the reduction of disease burden among the unvaccinated segment of a community in which a majority is immunised. Herd effect is indirect evidence that the vaccine has, in addition to individual protection, an effect on the transmission of the agent by immunised children, when they get infected after immunization. The respiratory route transmits all the four microbes mentioned above, and they multiply in the pharyngeal mucosa. The vaccines against them are inactivated products – in other words, completely non-infectious. All four vaccines are injected. Yet, they exhibit remarkable degrees of herd effect.

Herd effect is the epidemiologic or biologic consequence of mucosal protection. What is true of such injected vaccines seems to be a general phenomenon that is also applicable to IPV and poliovirus transmission.

Mucosal 'immunity' is induced only by local infection. Here there is no such 'immunity'. The lesson is: injected vaccines against diseases caused by mucosal infection are strong inducers of 'mucosal protection' that reduces the quantum and duration of the respiratory shedding of the microbe when the immune person is re-exposed. Reduction of quantum and duration of shedding of the microbe does not require mucosal 'immunity' but mucosal 'protection' resulting from high antibody levels in the blood. The same is true of IPV as well. IPV induces higher levels of polio antibodies than OPV. The mucosal protection required for the herd effect of all these respiratory transmitted agents is in the pharynx. IPV is a strong inducer of mucosal protection against polioviruses in the throat.

Human papilloma viruses are sexually transmitted. Mucosal protection is essential to prevent primary infection, as the chronicity of infection and risk of cervical cancer cannot be prevented after primary infection. An immunologically naïve way of thinking could be that we need a vaccine that is applied in the genital mucosa for predictable protection. Reality is that a non-infectious viral structural subunit vaccine is nearly 100 per cent efficacious in preventing infection. HPV vaccine provides sufficient mucosal protection without eliciting mucosal immunity. We cannot blame those who blindly believed in the paradigm of faecal-oral transmission of wild polioviruses and filled some gaps with unproven assumptions. The paradigm was handy to promote the live oral vaccine; belief in the vaccine and belief in the paradigm went hand in hand. But we could ask why they rejected all the evidences from many country experiences. Strong belief in the paradigm and the need to avoid cognitive dissonance could be the most plausible reason.

Summation

All evidences agree with the respiratory route of transmission of wild poliovirus, and none agrees with faecal-oral route of transmission. The only reason why the oral route is considered plausible is the fact that OPV is given by mouth and the vaccine viruses infect the intestines in some, but not all.

The very fact that the oral feeding of an unnaturally high inoculum dose of vaccine viruses fail to infect infants and children in many tropical low income countries with very low standards of hygiene and sanitation, and, requires an unreasonable number of inoculations for establishing gut infection, flies in the face of oral route of natural poliovirus infection. The fastest natural poliovirus transmission is in infants, when faecal contamination is least likely. The paradox is the ease of natural infection versus the difficulty for vaccine virus infection. These phenomena are associated with the very low hygiene and sanitation that leads to frequent infections with innumerable intestinal infections in infants and children. The reason for this association has not been elucidated.

The epidemiology of polio is nearly identical to that of measles, an undisputedly respiratory transmitted infection. What is striking is why so few people have concluded based on evidences that natural polio is respiratory transmitted. Such is the power of the belief in the paradigm of faecal-oral route of transmission. The predicament faced by the polio eradication program is the unfortunate result of that faith in the paradigm. A paradigm shift requires a threshold number of opinion leaders getting convinced of the anomalies in their paradigm.

The very purpose of this book is to advocate for that paradigm shift, which will enable the polio eradication program to accept evidence and reject dogma, and come on track to complete and conclude the program, satisfying ethics, epidemiology and economics of polio eradication.

§§§

7. PROOF OF PRINCIPLE AND COUNTRY MODELS

"Before embarking on a mega project involving huge investments, a wise investor will ascertain high probability of success and profit."

There are terms like proof of principle, proof of concept, proof of feasibility, pilot project, prototype, demonstration model etc. that are very relevant in the assessment of the likelihood of success in any large project, as in business or industry, so in public health.

Global level eradication of a disease is a mammoth project that would require enormous investments. Only if proof of principle is established and country-level model is available or pilot-tested, should anyone take courage, or have any moral right, to embark on global level disease eradication agenda. It is not to be undertaken light-heartedly or ill-advisedly.

If the disease had been deliberately eliminated from one or more countries using interventions, that information offers the necessary country model and proof of principle that the likelihood of success in other countries is extremely high. If

156

so, global eradication is feasible. The first country or countries that eliminated the disease will stand out as pilot projects or country models that have validated the proof of principle.

The first element of the proof of principle is predictable protection of individuals from disease by an intervention – in our case, with a vaccine. If the probability of individual protection with a vaccine is not very high – in other words, the efficacy of a vaccine is not near-100% after the recommended number of doses, that vaccine is not the ideal tool for elimination (country level), or, eradication (globally) of that disease. In the case of global polio eradication program, prescribing trivalent OPV with very low vaccine efficacy in tropical low income countries, as low as 10% per dose and 30% for 3 doses did not conform to the proof of principle and was contrary to conventional wisdom.

Smallpox was the first, and so far the only example of global level eradication of human disease; vaccination was effective to protect the vaccinated in the face of exposure to sick individuals with smallpox. Many countries in Europe, two in North America and also Japan had eliminated the indigenous transmission of smallpox, through widespread vaccination, long before the global eradication program was launched. Those countries were the models that gave public health leaders full confidence that smallpox could be globally eradicated, given the following: right ingredients of strategy, tactics and logistics of vaccination; and evidence-based monitoring to follow the trajectory of disease prevention and control, until eradication was achieved and verified.

Polio Eradication: Proof of Principle and Country Models

Proof of principle that polio could be prevented in the individual by immunization, controlled in the community by a successful immunization program, and, eliminated in a large population such as a whole country by sustained high coverage through the immunization program, had been available from the 1960s.

Five countries had eliminated the indigenous transmission of wild polioviruses using IPV – Finland, Sweden, Norway, The Netherlands and Iceland. As OPV was not used, there was no polio due to vaccine viruses -- VAPP in vaccinated or contact VAPP. All of them had high-quality public health surveillance that provided reliable data on the occurrence of any polio, and also adequate laboratory facilities to detect any poliovirus in any human subject with acute flaccid paralysis. These countries offered the country models of polio elimination, validating the proof of principle for global polio eradication.

The USA and several European countries had been using OPV in their national immunization programmes since the mid-1960s. The first element of proof of principle, namely the predictable protection of the vaccinated individual, was fulfilled in all these countries; OPV, given three times, was virtually 100% efficacious. USA, Germany and the UK were using OPV exclusively. France allowed both OPV and IPV in the national immunization program, and freedom was given to families and paediatricians to choose either.

All of these countries succeeded in eliminating wild virus transmission, but all of them had VAPP in small numbers. As elimination must result in zero polio, none of them had achieved true polio elimination status. They did not offer country models for polio elimination using only OPV.

Then in 1983, France introduced the new generation enhanced potency IPV developed in The Netherlands and France.[1] From 1984, there was no case of VAPP in France, as IPV coverage was high and OPV use on the decline. An occasional case of 'vaccine-failure polio' was a problem in France, but none had occurred since 1987 after OPV was discontinued.[1] Thus, France provided a second model of eliminating wild virus polio using both OPV and IPV and then eliminating vaccine-virus polio by increasing IPV coverage. We must add that the France model was not yet final in 1988 – the very last case of polio was in 1989. However, the lessons learned in France were clear and valid: wild virus polio could be eliminated using OPV and IPV, but polio elimination, including vaccine virus polio, required IPV.

Denmark was plagued with a very high incidence of polio in the 1930s through early 1950s. The country introduced IPV in 1955, locally manufactured in Copenhagen. The vaccination schedule was a dose each at 5, 6 and 15 months of age. After excellent control, a small outbreak of polio occurred in 1961, many of them were vaccine-failure cases. We quote Herdis von Magnus and Inger Petersen: "The vaccine failures can be ascribed to the low antigenicity of some vaccine batches during the first years of production and also to the intradermal inoculation technique used to stretch the limited amount of vaccine available."[2] In 1963, a nation-wide campaign was conducted to give monovalent OPV type 1 to all below 40 years without any untoward event. In 1966, another campaign was conducted with monovalent type 3 vaccine; five cases of paralytic polio occurred in close relation to vaccination. From 1967 trivalent OPV was introduced – now the vaccination schedule was IPV 3 doses as described above, followed by OPV 3 doses at 3, 4 and 5 years of age. Thereafter Denmark has remained with very few cases (one each in 1966, 1969 and 1980) and without any case since 1980.[2]

Denmark offered a model of using IPV and OPV in sequential schedules that achieved total polio elimination. As of 1988, these three were the only country-level models of polio elimination that offered the proof of principle that polio could be eradicated globally. Basically, all three showed that IPV was necessary for the design of the strategy and tactics of immunization for eradication.

The Danish model had some lessons for the Expanded Program on Immunization (EPI) – three doses of IPV followed by three doses of OPV could satisfy the desire to retain OPV in the eradication strategy for a short period. After reaching zero polio status, or after reaching the year 2000, whichever was earlier, OPV could be withdrawn without risk of polio due to emergence of VDPVs – or transmission if any VDPV had already emerged or was imported.

Deviating from these models and taking a different approach would not guarantee eradication – that would be very risky. The duty of the global polio eradication program was to upscale any of the three models, in partnership with member countries of the WHO. Deviating from proven models would be unfair to member countries and to the whole world.

What about proof of principle for OPV for polio eradication?

Although OPV by itself had not been successful in any country model to eliminate polio – hence proof of principle for polio eradication using OPV alone has never been validated, OPV was widely being used in many high-income countries as well as in all low-income countries that had adopted the EPI.

In high-income countries, OPV was highly efficacious in protecting children from wild virus polio. In almost all such countries wild polioviruses were eliminated, but VAPP (in vaccinated and in contacts) stood in the way of polio elimination. Thus the proof of principle was only that wild polioviruses could be eliminated with OPV, not that polio *per se* could be eliminated with OPV alone. The problem was the persistence of VAPP as long as OPV was used. Another problem was chronic vaccine poliovirus infection in immuno-deficient individuals who continued to shed vaccine-derived polioviruses that had regained neurovirulence. It was obvious that polio could not be eliminated with OPV alone.

Eventually, but not before the year of the resolution, 1988, all the rich countries that had eliminated wild polioviruses using OPV followed the France model and replaced OPV with IPV and thus eliminated polio altogether. Thus, in 1989 Germany switched from OPV to IPV and became the first country to create the model of 'OPV alone for wild virus elimination and IPV alone for vaccine virus elimination'. France had used both vaccines in the national immunization program and had given the choice of vaccine to paediatricians and families of children until the all-IPV schedule was implemented.[1]

The next country to switch from exclusive OPV to exclusive IPV was the USA. There were three years of transition – 1997, 1998 and 1999, in which both OPV and IPV were in use. Each year they also had small numbers of VAPP. USA provided further proof of principle that OPV was sufficient to eliminate wild polioviruses, but was incompatible with polio elimination. In 2000 USA eliminated polio under the exclusive use of IPV.

Thereafter Canada, New Zealand, UK, Ireland, Australia, Japan, many West European countries, South Korea, Taiwan, Brunei, Malaysia and a few more have followed that model. Currently, some 50 countries use IPV exclusively, and all of them have sustained their polio elimination status.

What about low-income countries that could not afford IPV?

The strength of a chain is as good as that of its weakest link. Numerically, weak links, low-income countries, by far outnumbered the strong and extra strong links. Eradication strategy and tactics had to be appropriate for success in all low-income countries.

Had there been no program to eradicate polio, the problem of choice between affordable OPV and unaffordable IPV could have been ducked, saying that it was almost catch-22. That was if the cost was the only consideration. What did not get due attention was ethics – we will present ethics appraisal in another chapter.

However, the cost dilemma changed drastically in 1988, with the WHA Resolution for global polio eradication by 2000. Eradication was the goal, irrespective of the cost – lower the better. Also, time was short – the progressive decline in polio due to wild viruses and the avoidance of VAPP had to be rather rapidly and convincingly shown to the world – to the munificent donors, the bewildered low-income countries, the public health leaders of all countries and the media everywhere. Only twelve years were available for the program. However, WHO had a great advantage and unusual opportunity – to focus attention on the three Regions of South-East Asia, Africa and Eastern Mediterranean. Instead, WHO chose to work with the three Regions that had resolved on their own to eliminate polio by or before 2000 – Americas, Europe and Western Pacific – thereby dissipating professional time, efforts and money simply to make sure one size fitted all.

The situation was very serious, challenging and complicated and deserved careful 'war room' planning and weighing out war strategies, choice of tactics – and how to use the available weapons of war to the best advantage – quick victory, least collateral damage and lowest cost. Country models were already available for clear guidance. The merits of both vaccines and a comparison of their efficacy and safety were described in the third and fourth chapters.

Today, in 2019-2020, the program has only the exact opposites to show to the world – no victory yet in sight after 31-32 years. Also, too much collateral damage by way of program-caused polio outnumbering wild virus polio annually for a decade and about a billion US dollars spent every year for the past 19-20 years. War room planning apparently had not taken place; if it had taken place, it was hidden from public view and also, obviously, grossly flawed. The real reason for deviating from proven country models has never been explicit --could the reason have been in the mind's 'affective' domain (with beliefs and biases) and not in the 'cognitive' domain (with logic, reasoning and guidance from country models)?

The first element of proof of principle was not fulfilled with OPV, as children developed wild virus polio despite 3, 4, 5, 7, 10 and even more doses of OPV. In other words, OPV, given in a reasonably acceptable number of doses, did not predictably prevent polio. The efficacy of OPV was very low. It was hardly fit as a weapon in this war, let alone the only weapon. The deliberate choice of the less fit or unfit weapon makes us strongly suspect that the reason was irrational, hence in the affective domain of the minds of the program experts.

One could argue that the efficacy of OPV was low but not zero; hence it could be built upon. Yes, indeed, but too many doses are required. That would not only delay eradication but also jack up the cost of the program -- the cost of vaccine and cost of vaccine administration. Five doses in EPI and annually two national-level campaigns for all under-five children as done in India for many years had add up to 15 doses by age 5.

Even, so there was no promise of success – only a gamble, not wise in war. Moreover, vaccine failure polio would occur in unacceptable numbers, since polio was predominantly in children under two years who would not be fully protected as they could not be given the needed 15 doses. Full protection by five years of age was not early enough.

What the generous donors to the program did not realise, was, that one OPV campaign, very likely, cost as much as what one dose of IPV for all children would have cost. As for IPV, 2 or 3 doses of IPV would have been sufficient to fully protect. Children could be fully protected even in the first year of life. Therefore, obviously, the cost of eradication using IPV would have been very much lower than attempting to eradicate using too many repeated campaigns of OPV. The time needed for eradication could have been drastically cut short.

If eradication had to be completed by the year 2000, enhanced potency IPV had to be introduced in EPI earlier than later. Five years of preparation from 1988 would have been sufficient for universal introduction of IPV. In 1993 IPV in EPI could be topped up with OPV either in EPI or by a limited number of campaigns. As IPV coverage was built up, many countries would have eliminated polio, and in them, OPV could be withdrawn. This was the most reasonable strategy as of 1988, with the available proof of principle and successful country models. Moreover, IPV supply could be up-scaled as demand increased, and cost of production reduced with the improvements in production technology perfected in the early 1980s in The Netherlands and in France.

This approach was most probably in the vision of those who drafted the WHA Resolution, stipulating that eradication be achieved through EPI and using vaccines – which could have only meant both vaccines – OPV and IPV.

What the eradication program leaders took rather as a mere choice between two vaccines, OPV and IPV – was, in reality, the choice between eradication through EPI and eradication through a new global vertical program.[3] IPV is the truly EPI-friendly vaccine, necessary and sufficient in 2-3 doses, given in combination with other injected EPI vaccines due simultaneously, whereas OPV, necessary in many more doses than the number of contacts of health workers with children, turned out to be not EPI-friendly at all. The program had a choice between adopting the proven models with a higher chance of success and experimenting with the unproven strategy of the exclusive use of OPV that required repeated doses in the same children, for which repeated community campaigns and even house-to-house campaigns were necessary.

What lessons from the eradication of wild virus type 2?

Among the three types of viruses in trivalent OPV, type 2 was far more efficacious than types 1 and 3. That was clearly proved in Vellore in the late 1960s and early 1970s. That important fact was confirmed in the eradication program, as wild type 2 polio was eradicated in 1999, one year ahead of the target of 2000 for polio eradication.

If one type of wild virus could be eradicated using trivalent OPV, did that not offer proof of principle that the other two types also could be eradicated using trivalent OPV? Yes, and No. If in the middle of the war, no; just one year was left to finish the war and the fact that only one type was eradicated meant failure with types 1 and 3.

If the eradication program was not on, there would not have been an awful hurry, and there would have been some time to test out how the game could be played out.

Eradication of wild type 2 was also clear evidence that tOPV coverage had reached an optimum level. It was also clear evidence that vaccine efficacies of types 1 and 3 components were utterly insufficient for eradicating them using tOPV, even with optimum coverage. The program persisting with the same weapon to fight the war on polio was indicative of very disturbing attitude or mindset of the program managers, which we attributed to psychological 'path-fixation' – not knowing how and when to change tactics and weapons.

There was no War General with accountability to a higher authority, unlike in the case of the smallpox eradication program. The style of functioning seemed as if some committee was in charge – or some committees. There was no war room review and critical assessment of, or intelligent modification of, the war tactics and weapon usage. The choice, of exclusive use of OPV, and the exclusion of IPV, was contrary to evidence and reasoning – it was irrational. The real meaning of eradication of type 2 wild virus was not appreciated – the program apparently chose to believe that if one type could be eradicated the other types also could be eradicated. That was neither logical nor realistic -- but most unwise, bordering on foolhardy. History has proved it to be so. What we see clearly in hindsight ought to have been foreseen by program experts, had they been true experts with expertise and depth of knowledge.

In the USA, when OPV was introduced in the national immunization program in the 1960s, VAPP appeared and paralysed many children – showing OPV's safety problem. What happened then was not a wise, compassionate, logical, realistic, ethical decision, but what was provided was a strong defence of the earlier wrong decision. Another example of not knowing how to change a decision made just a few years earlier? In other words, 'path fixation'?

We say wrong boldly since IPV was re-introduced in 1996 and OPV was abandoned in 2000 – clearly showing that the OPV-only choice was wrong. Top-level decision-makers tend not to admit errors of judgment, but instead, they tend to vehemently justify their earlier 'wrong' decisions with strong (not necessarily valid) arguments.

We have heard some saying that 1996 was not 1966; conditions had drastically changed'. False logic; polioviruses have not changed behaviour. Your ability to predict what polioviruses will or will not do is proportional to your expertise and experience with polio in the community.

In 1966, the USA was ready to stop smallpox vaccination as the risk from vaccination far outweighed the benefit from protection – there was no more smallpox in the North American Continent. But smallpox vaccination was causing serious adverse reactions in some individuals. Medical and public health science had effective means to screen people travelling to USA and Canada and ensure that travellers did not import smallpox; in case someone did bring in smallpox, intervention protocol was ready. Unfortunately, public health experts dealing with smallpox vaccination and polio vaccination were not the same people.

We must distinguish between 'excuses' from 'reasons'. Persisting with OPV had many excuses, but not any valid reasons. Eventually, in 1996, the old excuses evaporated, good sense and wisdom prevailed – USA introduced IPV and after three years abandoned OPV altogether.

The France-Germany model was absolutely valid. Think of the time delay – nearly three decades. Think of the collateral damage – about 300 paralysed people.[4]

The global polio eradication program did not quite grasp these stark realities even in the year 2000 when it realised that wild virus type 2 had stopped circulating any everywhere.

Lessons from the eradication of type 3 wild poliovirus

Type 2 wild poliovirus was globally eradicated in 1999 as we saw earlier. That was proof enough that types 1 and 3 wild polioviruses could not be eradicated with the same vaccine that achieved type 2 eradication, namely trivalent OPV (tOPV) – the mixture of vaccine virus strains of types 1, 2 and 3. What next? There was clear evidence from various studies that type 2 was dominant in tOPV and that it interfered with immune response to types 1 and 3.

In 2002, three years after the last case of type 2 wild virus polio in the world, there was no more need for the type 2 strain in the vaccine – if type 2 was removed, the resultant bivalent OPV (bOPV) had a better chance of eradicating types 1 and 3 wild viruses. Immediate research to compare the vaccine efficacy of bOPV and tOPV against types 1 and 3 polioviruses would have settled the question – but that was not done in the next five years. Eventually it was done, but precious time was lost. Was the problem a total reluctance, emotionally, to admit that one strain in OPV was now undesirable, thereby admitting that OPV was not the perfect vaccine that the experts were telling everyone?

Where the vaccine efficacy of trivalent OPV (tOPV) was very low against types 1 and 3, monovalent OPV (mOPV) had two-and-a-half times higher efficacy.[5] By 2005-2006, mOPV type 1 and mOPV type 3 were introduced into the program. Then bOPV – types 1 and 3 without type 2 – was investigated and found to be non-inferior to monovalent vaccines. But when was this information available to the program leaders? The head-to-head comparison of monovalent and trivalent OPVs had been published in a paper in the Bulletin of the WHO in 1976.[5] Only in 2005, it was re-validated, in Egypt and in India, when it was obvious that wild virus polio will not be eradicated using tOPV.[6,7] Even in 2005, the eradication program experts were unwilling to remove type 2 from OPV, in spite of evidence that it would have enhanced the protective efficacy of the other two components. Science and logic were not guiding the program experts.

Vaccination coverage sufficient to create of near-100 per cent immunity was recognised as required for interrupting transmission of types 1 and 3 polioviruses, no less. Also, many repeated doses were required to increase vaccine efficacy. So, in India for example, children in schools, those travelling in buses and trains, children in migrant labour camps and in difficult-to-reach communities were identified and reached. The wild virus type 3 was eradicated in 2012 using all the above approaches. That was 13 long years after type 2 had been eradicated in 1999. What should have been obvious to experts was finally proven – trivalent OPV would not have eradicated type 3 wild poliovirus at all. Defenders of the war tactics would say: we won – but at what financial cost, with what human price and with what time delay?

What about the original target of the year 2000? By 2001, the knotty problem of two outbreaks of circulating vaccine-derived polioviruses (cVDPVs) one with type 2 (in Egypt) in the 1980s and the other with type 1 (in Haiti and Dominican Republic in the Caribbean island of Hispaniola,) in 2000 became widely recognised. But the eradication program did not understand the sinister significance of these signals. With persistent use of OPV, there have been too many outbreaks of polio due to vaccine-derived viruses in several countries every year since 2005. In 2019 there were such outbreaks in 19 countries and in 2020 in 25 countries.

The Resolution's stipulations were not respected

Proof of principle and precedents are of crucial importance in designing large public health programmes. Before 1988 there was sufficient data to to show that wild polioviruses would not be eliminated using OPV through EPI in low-income countries in the tropical zone. As pointed out earlier, vaccine efficacy of trivalent OPV was unsatisfactorily low in many low-income countries in the tropical zone around the world.

OPV by campaigns had been experimented in Brazil and in Vellore town in South India, and in both locations, the incidence of polio declined drastically. The campaign approach was called national immunization days (NIDs) in Brazil and in other countries in South America. It was called 'pulse immunization' in Vellore.[8] With two annual national immunization days Brazil was able to drastically reduce polio incidence. With three pulse polio campaigns at monthly intervals, Vellore town was able to reach zero polio status. These provided proof of principle that OPV had to be de-linked from EPI schedule, and given in annual pulse immunization or NIDs, for the purpose of eliminating wild polioviruses.

The resolution wanted polio eradication achieved through EPI. OPV through EPI was not sufficient to eradicate wild polioviruses in low-income countries. Moreover, because of the risk of VAPP, OPV was incompatible with polio elimination in low-income countries, as in high-income countries.

Achieving the polio eradication goal clearly required introduction and ramping up of IPV and ramping down of OPV – exclusive OPV through EPI was clearly not sufficient. The resolution had recognised that polio vaccines should be used. We believe that the experts who drafted the resolution had seen the possibility or the potential of IPV in polio eradication strategy and tactics. Moreover, proof of principle is invaluable in scaling up a project, and there was no justification to ignore it and put the project in jeopardy.

Summation

No country ever had eliminated polio, caused by both wild polioviruses and Sabin strains of vaccine polioviruses, without achieving high coverage of IPV. OPV can only eliminate wild polioviruses. IPV is necessary to eliminate vaccine polioviruses.[9] These simple facts had been shown by country models of polio elimination much before the WHA Resolution was drafted in 1988. The reason why the global polio eradication program ignored the available proof of principle and country models and insisted on an OPV-only policy for polio eradication could not have been ignorance of facts but some unknown factor that seemed to have over-ruled science and reality. That is why we suggest that biases were involved. Biases are, in general, hidden from the cognitive domain of the mind.

Sometimes a clever war strategy, different from what proof of principle had shown, could be justified if it leads to quick victory with minimum collateral damage and reasonable financial cost. The OPV-only strategy has not stood that test of justification.

§§§

Section Three

Global polio eradication is a gargantuan public health program that started with great hope, unprecedented international cooperation, robust science, cutting edge technology, generous funding. Two vaccines that promised success if used for best human advantage, with science, ethics and wisdom, without dogma clouding evidence, without personal preferences and biases, would have achieved the desired result on time. The destination was defined incorrectly as a world without wild-virus polio, with vaccine-caused polio condoned as trivial adverse reaction to live virus vaccine but not as polio. Untruth repeated by a thousand people a thousand times does not become truth. Truth, if held by a minority, even if a minority of two, however inconvenient, is still truth – truth to be told to the thousand people and to the whole world. Global polio eradication is still achievable if vaccine-caused polio is defined as polio that must also be eradicated.

8. ETHICS AND POLIO ERADICATION

"Relativity applies to physics, not ethics." Albert
Einstein

*"It is a paradox that medical experimentation on individuals,
whether patients or healthy volunteers, is now controlled by
strict ethical guidelines, while no such protection exists for
whole populations which are subjected to medical interventions
in the name of preventive medicine or health promotion."* Petr
Scrabanek

Ethics in Health Management

Ethics represents concepts and knowledge concerned with
moral principles that govern a person's behaviour or activity,
especially when it affects other persons. Medical ethics guides
healthcare personnel in their transactions with patients and
their families -- to understand what is morally right or wrong,
in specific contexts.

Health management, using modern scientific medicine, consists of 'public health', 'healthcare' and 'biomedical research' – the last one for constant improvement of the former two. Ethics is strictly enforced in all medical research. Every research study proposal and plan have to go through a thorough review by a properly established Institutional Review Board (IRB): approval by the IRB is mandatory.

Healthcare is 'clinical medicine' (diagnosis, therapeutics, surgery, rehabilitation) which includes 'preventive medicine' (screening for risk factors or for early detection of diseases before they manifest and their mitigation and need-based vaccinations). In healthcare medical ethics guides all decisions as applied to patients. The declaration of Human Rights by the United Nations had made it clear that sick persons seeking healthcare -- weak and vulnerable as they may be, have human rights that have to be ensured during all transactions. The core fundamental principles of healthcare ethics were framed by Tom Beauchamp and James Childress in the 1970s.[1]

These are:

1.   Non-maleficence (do no harm),
2.   Beneficence (act for the benefit and well-being of the other party).
3.   Justice (equitably distribute benefits, risks, costs, and resources) and
4.   Autonomy (respect for individual's right for making an informed decision).

Ethics in vaccination as preventive medicine

Vaccines undergo rigorous screening before they are licensed in various countries. The first vaccine to be licensed against rotavirus diarrhoea, a live virus vaccine with the trade name Rotashield, was manufactured and marketed by a company in the USA in August 1998. Although it was highly effective against rotavirus diarrhoea, in the post-marketing phase it was found to be associated with an unexpected adverse reaction – an increase in the occurrence of a rare but serious childhood disease called intussusception -- a segment of the intestine telescoping into itself, the upper portion into the lower portion. Blood supply to the affected portion gets blocked, resulting in tissue death that is called necrosis in medical language. When a portion of intestine has necrosis the intestinal contents spill out into the sterile space around, and that triggers a series of events that leads to death. Prompt diagnosis and treatment are life-saving. This safety problem, namely a slight increase in intussusceptions cases following Rotashield vaccination, was detected in USA through a surveillance method called the 'Vaccine Adverse Events Reporting System'.

Here was a conundrum. The cause of intussusception is unknown and natural (wild) rotaviruses do not cause it. So, could a rotavirus vaccine cause intussusception? Probably not -- at least in the strict sense of the causality principle of evidence-based cause-and-effect. So, the vaccine seems to be "triggering" the occurrence of intussusception. The child with it now, would not have developed it, if vaccine had not been given.

The company withdrew the vaccine from market, in October 1999, fourteen months after its licensure. The overall benefit-to-risk assessment of the vaccine was actually good: the vaccine would avert many more severe cases of rotavirus disease, hospitalization and deaths than those due to the rare adverse reaction. But, transferring risks from some to others contravenes ethics – specifically non-maleficence. That is why the company voluntarily withdrew the vaccine from market. Supporting that decision, the Advisory Committee on Immunization Practices (ACIP) of the US Centers for Disease Control and Prevention (CDC) withdrew its recommendation of routine immunization of infants with Rotashield vaccine.[3] Ethics does not approve benefit to many at the cost of a few. Subsequently, safe live virus vaccines against rotavirus diarrhoea have been developed and are in use in many countries.

Until 1980, the vaccine against rabies was prepared by growing rabies virus in the brains of animals – sheep, goats, rabbits, suckling mice – and completely inactivating with chemicals. While such vaccines were highly effective in preventing rabies when given soon after bite of rabid animals, and very affordable in low income countries where rabies kills many, there was a safety problem with it, due to the animal brain-tissue in the vaccine. Very occasionally, vaccine recipients developed a neurological illness, often causing limb paralysis, mostly self-limited with full recovery – but not always. Very rarely death ensued. In benefit-risk assessment, benefit far outweighed risk – rabies was always fatal. Even cost-effectiveness was excellent. But medical ethics demanded the development of a completely safe vaccine and by 1980 such safe rabies vaccine made in cell culture became available, and the animal brain rabies vaccine was eventually withdrawn or disallowed in all countries. Ethics over-ruled economic advantage. Ethics also demanded development of safe rabies vaccine without serious adverse reaction to the dog-bite victims.

Economic assessment allows choice related to products – cheaper the better, but ethics is non-compromising, non-negotiable. When two products for one purpose are available but one does not satisfy the tenets of medical ethics, it should be withdrawn or disallowed. If it is not withdrawn, countries making autonomous decisions should disallow it in their citizens.

Vaccination has been at the eye of the storm for a long time, in the field of medical ethics. Ethical issues are inherent right from the stages of vaccine research, it's licensing for human use, and its prescription for individuals by healthcare staff. Vaccines are meant to benefit by protecting the vaccinated individuals, mostly children, against target diseases. Sometimes a conflict may emerge between the need to get vaccinated for individual benefit (protection from disease) and the need or opportunity to get vaccinated for the benefit of family members who are vulnerable or of the community in general, by way of reduction of disease frequency. Ethics of vaccination of individuals with COVID-19 vaccines is widely recognized and highly relevant in all countries. In a disease control program, which is actually public health, the benefit to the community gets accentuated when many individuals are vaccinated. Public health ethics in vaccination is discussed later in this chapter.

Drugs against life-threatening diseases may be toxic, but ethics applies benefit-risk equation for the choice. Between the consequences of disease and drug, risk and benefit have to be carefully weighed. If life will be saved by toxic drugs, tolerating drug toxicity is the better choice – the lesser evil. But on the other hand, risks associated with the use of vaccines gain importance in ethics since healthy children or adults are involved.

If a vaccine is known to cause serious adverse reaction, its choice is based on benefit-risk analysis and the decision rests on the best interests of the individual. We clarified this question, illustrating with rabies vaccination in individuals bitten by dogs that may carry rabies virus in their saliva. When safe rabies vaccine became available the use of animal brain vaccine became unethical.

In a healthcare facility, the individual, child, adolescent or adult, is offered information by the physician or nurse about the vaccines that are available to protect them from specific infectious diseases. There is one to one discussion between the two parties. The benefits, and any risks involved with the administration of the vaccine, will be the essence of the discussion. In the case of children, parent or guardian stands in on the child's behalf. Here the individual's choice and decision to comply with the physician's advice is autonomous. The healthcare provider is bound by the Beauchamp-Childress principles, and codes of ethical conduct laid by the national agencies that prescribe and ensure ethical healthcare practice, such as national Medical Councils.

The choice made by the individual is for oneself, seldom based on the social responsibility of providing benefit to society. Here, it may be deemed unacceptable to the parent if the child suffers from adverse effects, the risk of which may outweigh the benefit the vaccine was meant to provide. Think of India, with wild virus polio eliminated (in 2011) and so certified (in 2014), continuing to vaccinate children with OPV that causes VAPP in some children. Causing polio with vaccine while natural polio has been eliminated surely raises serious ethical questions. So, many parents demand the safe poliovaccine, IPV. Pediatricians respect the autonomy of parents and vaccinate their children with IPV. The Indian Academy of Pediatrics recommends full immunizing course with IPV in the best interests of the children.

Ethics and the choice of vaccine against polio in EPI

The Expanded Program on Immunization (EPI) was launched by the WHO in 1974. There were then more than 100 countries without formal public health department or universal healthcare to ensure that all children got the benefit of immunization; EPI was critically important for them.

In countries with public health and universal access to healthcare, vaccines were, and are, provided in clinics in which a doctor or nurse interacts with the parents as described above. In such situations the public health policy on the use of vaccines in the control of diseases will be an additional item for discussion. Parents ought to know that the child's vaccination has community benefits to keep diseases under control. In such countries the quantitative measurements of disease burden are in the public domain in real-time and the choice of parents will include such objective data. Parents have the right of refusal but if refusals jeopardize the disease control program, that should be explicitly presented to the parents. In some countries full vaccination may be a requirement for school admission. In such countries the public health department would have included a vaccine only if ethical appraisal is positive. This is illustrated by some 50 countries with public health and universal access to healthcare, that have deemed OPV unethical and do not allow its use and IPV is made available to all children.

In countries adopting EPI, trained health workers, not well-versed with all aspects and details of the diseases and their vaccines, as well as the principles of ethics, vaccinate children according to a schedule made by the Government through its ministry of health. Health ministries of such countries are expected to make decisions in the best interests of individual children and the community at large – and within norms of ethics. Families trust the health workers who themselves are accountable only for the quality of service and strict adherence to prescribed protocols, but not for ethical propriety of vaccine choice. That trust emanates from their faith in the governments – that they will not mandate anything unethical. Thus governments have the duty to be honest and careful in the application of ethical principles.[2]

That duty was compromised in India, as it would have been in many other countries, quite contrary to the ethical principles of beneficence and non-maleficence. Right through 1970s, 1980s and 1990s medical fraternity, teachers of social and preventive medicine, teachers and students of public health would have read the many publications highlighting the efficacy problems of OPV. Many children, given the recommended number of doses of OPV, 3 or 4 or 5, were not protected from polio. Not taking action against that ethical problem surely contravened the principle of beneficence. What was true in India was true in many other countries. The most likely explanation for this problem is that ethics was not taught to be, or thought to be, important in health management.

Since EPI policies, choice of vaccines and schedules are provided to member countries by the WHO, it was essential that such recommendations are cleared for ethical healthcare and public health. However, the role of WHO is only recommendatory. The responsibility to adapt the recommendations to the citizens and their families is the responsibility of the country governments. Both agencies should have applied ethical assessment of their policy decisions – but did they do so? Do they make ethical assessments now?

EPI originally included vaccines against primary tuberculosis (BCG), diphtheria, pertussis, tetanus (DPT), measles and polio. The measles vaccine is a live virus vaccine, universally documented to be safe from serious adverse reactions and highly efficacious against measles disease. BCG and DPT, similarly, were known to be safe from serious adverse reactions. Now BCG is known not to be completely safe in children with HIV infection – EPI belongs to the pre-HIV era. At present, EPI does not recommend BCG in children known to be HIV infected for obvious ethical reasons -- a rare child may develop a serious disease due to the live organisms in BCG. Here ethics has precedence over risk-benefit evaluation.

For protection from polio, two vaccines were available – OPV and IPV. EPI recommended OPV exclusively, and all countries adopting EPI accepted it. No option was provided for a choice between the two vaccines which went against the ethics principle of autonomy. On account of the exclusion of IPV from EPI, the vaccine regulatory agency did not register IPV in India until 2006. The issues of safety and efficacy were not discussed with parents in EPI vaccination sessions. Also it was repeatedly said by EPI leaders and health workers that OPV was completely safe, an untruth, hence unethical. Was EPI for the best interests of individual children or collectively for the community? There was tension between the two that was not addressed by EPI. Ethics was not applied in EPI, to the best of our assessment.

Best interests of individuals and the community are two sides of the same coin: what is not in the best interests of the individual cannot be in the best interests of the community. Under the then given conditions, EPI was very important to protect the health and lives of children *en masse* in all WHO member countries without universal healthcare. For pragmatic and ethical reasons, there was justification for promoting EPI, since not vaccinating children against the six target diseases would have been unethical then – between vaccinating and not vaccinating, non-vaccination would have been highly unethical. The adoption of EPI in countries was a governmental decision; governments, especially democracies, are the best advocates of health promotion and disease prevention of all citizens and their families, and, decisions are expected to be *bona fide* and not *mala fide* or without diligent consideration. Once medical ethics became widely understood, medical colleges included is as a subject for didactic teaching, not applying ethics in EPI cannot be simply condoned.

When it came to polio prevention, there was a real choice between OPV and IPV. Both WHO and country governments had to follow ethical principles when faced with such a choice between two vaccines with starkly contrasting profiles of safety and efficacy. Here we will apply the four core principles of medical ethics for the choice between OPV and IPV.

a) Non-maleficence

Non-maleficence is equivalent to the age-old dictum, in Latin, *"Primum non nocere"* (first of all, do no harm) - it refers to the moral obligation to not allow harm, when providing a solution to a given problem – and to select harmless choice as against a potentially harmful choice, if such choice was available.

In 1957, AMM Payne, Chief in the Division of Communicable Diseases, WHO, had cautioned about the possibility of reversion to virulence of the vaccine virus in the individual's gut such viruses in the environment due to shedding of vaccine-viruses.[3]

Prophetic. That was before OPV was licensed in any country in the world. In the promotion of OPV by WHO, both in EPI and in polio eradication, Payne's caution had to be taken seriously and acted accordingly. The very first action required was verification. Payne's prediction, based on the then available information to WHO, had to be verified and proven wrong before OPV was chosen for exclusive use in EPI first and in polio eradication later.

In 1962, polio was detected in children given OPV (monovalent type 3) in the USA. In the following years, types 1 and 2 vaccines were also introduced and polio in children vaccinated with any vaccine virus type and particularly with the combination of all three, trivalent OPV, was too obvious to be neglected. In 1964, a special committee evaluated the matter and concluded that OPV was indeed causing polio and called this serious adverse reaction as VAPP. [4]

The WHO Committee on Poliomyelitis also investigated the problem in European countries and confirmed VAPP in all countries using OPV and also the safety (absence of VAPP) of IPV in countries using IPV.[5,6]

As we stated elsewhere in this book, OPV in EPI could have been justified for a limited period, if its intention was to rapidly control polio – that was not what happened. Did the lower cost of OPV than IPV – in other words, economic advantage – justify the exclusive use of OPV? As EPI was initiated, OPV could have been justified if it was for a limited period, with a plan to increase the use of IPV and a sunset plan to wind down the use of OPV. However, between economics and ethics, ethics ought to have been given greater value.

Research should have been conducted to minimise the cost of IPV production and to design a vaccination schedule to minimise the number of doses for optimal protection; these were required if the choice of OPV over IPV was based only on cost-considerations. Indeed such research was done, not in USA (the country of origin) but in Bilthoven in The Holland [7] and in Vellore in India.[8,9] but the results remained unutilized by EPI.[10]

In summary, the choice of the exclusive use of OPV in EPI did not satisfy the ethical principle of non-maleficence.

b) Beneficence

For beneficence, the vaccine should be able to predictably prevent paralysis due to wild poliovirus with high probability. Both OPV and IPV had proved to be highly efficacious in the USA and other high-income countries and to cause a substantial decrease in wild virus poliomyelitis, qualifying for beneficence in such countries.

But there was a major problem elsewhere. Soon after its introduction in low-income countries, there were reports of low seroconversion rates (i.e. low frequency of antibody responses, hence immunogenicity that reflects protective efficacy) following OPV, and also the occurrence of vaccine-failure polio cases as the corollary of low seroconversion rates. Many children given the recommended number of doses of OPV remained unprotected and developed polio – not milder polio but polio of the same severity as in unvaccinated children. For example, by 1987, (one year prior to the drafting of the WHA Resolution to eradicate polio), about half of all cases of polio in India were in children with a history of 3 doses of OPV – they were cases of polio due to vaccine-failure. On the other hand, IPV had been proved to induce immunity uniformly in infants, even with just two doses in rich and poor countries.

The reason for the difference in seroconversion frequencies and consequent occurrence of polio in large proportions of vaccinated children in low-income countries was not clear. All polio experts, globally, were aware of the low efficacy, but those in policy-making positions ignored it. It was postulated that there might be some inhibitors in the saliva and alimentary tract to infection by attenuated vaccine virus strains.[10]

The first report of 3-dose trivalent OPV-failure and resultant wild-virus polio in 'fully vaccinated' children according to EPI norms came from India, that too some years before the launch of EPI.[11] Ironically, the definitive studies confirming this 'infirmity' of OPV were conducted at the behest of WHO, well before EPI was launched. The non-utilisation of WHO-sponsored research findings that OPV had unacceptably low vaccine efficacy remains unexplained – but it clearly showed gross bias in favour of OPV and neglect of the values of both science and ethics.

Families who trusted the EPI and received just three doses of OPV but still developed polio were unfortunate victims of the exclusive use of OPV in EPI. The trust was not rewarded with full protection, grossly unfair to children.

In summary, the choice of the exclusive use of OPV did not satisfy the ethics principle of beneficence in many countries adopting EPI.

c) Autonomy

Decision-makers usually believe they are the best judges in the contextual need for a decision. All sides of the issue ought to be available to them to make such decisions. Those who are least informed and/or pressurised by others are often incapable of autonomous decisions. Yet a decision is needed. To protect children from polio, it may be assumed that various governments had made a procedurally autonomous decision, not what was recommended by international or United Nations agencies such as WHO or UNICEF, and, with complete understanding of what is best for their children.

But there appears to be no evidence of discussions with scientists /researchers for the choice of a vaccine in low-income countries. No such discussion has been divulged in the public domain. In India we know that such discussion has not taken place and many scientific reports in medical journals have not made any impact on the decision-making process. Consequently the immunization policies of Indian Academy of Pediatrics and India EPI (called Universal Immunization Program, UIP) are contradictory and the tension remains unresolved over decades. The Academy recommends full immunizing schedule of IPV for children, while accommodating the UIP recommendation of OPV also. The UIP recommendation is a replica of the WHO EPI recommendation. There is no opportunity for informed consent by the parents to be able to take an autonomous decision to choose between OPV and IPV. The parents/guardians are obliged to accept the polio vaccine offered under UIP. Thus, the choice of the exclusive use of OPV did not satisfy the autonomy principle.

In the case of India, as in many other countries, the national regulatory agency did not allow the entry of IPV from 1974 until IPV was licensed. In India IPV was licensed for use in the private sector in 2006 for the first time, apparently as the regulatory agency was convinced of the safety and efficacy of IPV. As far as we know that decision was on its own accord and not in response to application by any vaccine company.

In 2015 the polio eradication program and WHO declared that in 2016 type 2 component of trivalent OPV would be withdrawn and tOPV replaced by bOPV containing only types 1 and 3. That vaccine- switch was fraught with some risks and for risk-mitigation one dose of IPV was required for all children who would be offered bOPV. For that reason IPV was licensed in all countries that were using OPV until then. Once licensed, IPV became very popular in the private sector in India, and in many other countries as well. The Indian Academy of Pediatrics made IPV as its formal policy. The availability of both vaccines in countries using the EPI schedule vitiates the next principle of ethics – justice. However it is good that IPV has been licensed in all countries.

d) Justice

The principle of justice is the moral obligation to choose fairly – meaning, with the best interests of the recipient party -- between competing claims – in our case between two vaccines.

What is fair? Equity and equality are implicit in fairness and justice. EPI was designed to provide equal opportunities for all children, irrespective of their circumstances, to get vaccinated against the six diseases. That was laudable, exemplary.

However, in the choice between OPV and IPV, the principle of justice was already compromised in that children in rich countries got the safe IPV while children in low-income countries had to accept OPV with its low efficacy and incomplete safety. The problem was amplified in many low-income countries in which IPV was licensed: children of rich families had access to IPV in the private sector, while children who availed the government sector immunization program were forced to be satisfied with OPV. The ethical principle of justice was indeed compromised.

Summary

We, as paediatricians, always conscious of the best interests and welfare of all children we care for, have been uncomfortable with the policy of exclusive use of OPV while the safe and effective IPV was available in the global market. Had IPV not been available, the use of OPV would have been ethically acceptable because benefit-risk would have favoured immunization with the available vaccine. That was like using animal brain rabies vaccine to prevent rabies. No alternate vaccine was available until the third quarter of the twentieth century. Once safe cell culture vaccines became available, the animal brain vaccines became ethically unacceptable according to the Beuchamp-Childress principles. The availability of two vaccines against polio imposed the responsibility of choice on decision-makers in authority – and that choice had to satisfy the four elements in healthcare ethics.

We must remember that up until 1988 and the eradication resolution, the sole purpose of EPI was to prevent polio in individual children. There was no polio control program in vogue, as evidenced by the absence of a polio surveillance system – the two interventions for disease control are surveillance and vaccination program. Under those circumstances the choice of OPV for exclusive use clearly contravened the four ethical principles.

How disturbingly true is the observation: "It is a paradox that medical experimentation on individuals, whether patients or healthy volunteers, is now controlled by strict ethical guidelines , while no such protection exist for whole populations which are subjected to medical interventions in the name of preventive medicine or health promotion."[11]

***

Public Health Ethics and Polio Eradication

Disease eradication is a global level public health program. Public health has nothing personal in applying biomedical interventions in people, unlike in preventive medicine in healthcare.

Eradication results in the removal of a pathogen from all countries, without changing the socioeconomic disparities between countries. The resultant benefit of the absence of disease is enjoyed by all, providing absolute equity in that one specific context. Public health is thus for equity, all sharing benefits and risks equally. Therefore, public health has a moral obligation to ensure that risks, if any, are also shared equally. In other words, no one, or no specific group, should have any more risk than anyone else, when some risk is involved − risk should be randomly distributed. Disturbingly that has not been the case with the polio eradication program.

The principles of healthcare ethics alone may not suffice to make ethical decisions for a public health program where the subjects concerned are members of the community, not specifically identified individuals. Public health ethics encompasses some broader issues which include fundamentality, interdependence and community trust.

It may be argued that policymakers had applied the moral principle of "Utilitarianism" which means being morally right if the action leads to "greater good for greater number" even if harmful to a few. In contrast, "Deontology" respects fundamental rights of all, and, prohibits any wrong even to a minority. In Utilitarianism, the consequence of action matters while in Deontology the morality of action matters more than the just consequence. The program leaders may argue that the use of OPV was in line with the principle of Utilitarianism, where the greater outcome of polio eradication could ignore the adverse effects that the program had caused in a minority. On the other hand, OPV will not qualify for Deontology, considering its safety problems. Utilitarianism would have easily overruled Deontology if OPV was the only one available to the world or if OPV had succeeded in the mission of global polio eradication by 2000. Neither clause saves the situation. Polio could not be eradicated by 2000. The availability of a totally safe and more efficacious IPV settles fairly and squarely the ethics case against OPV.

Seven ethical principles for public health immunization

In 2012, David Isaacs proposed seven ethical principles for a public heath immunization program to be ethically justifiable. These principles are: Benefits, Risks, Effectiveness, Equity and justice, Autonomy, Reciprocity and Trust as discussed below.[12]

1) Benefits

The program should benefit the individual and community.

In preventive medicine under healthcare, only the individual gets to benefit from vaccination. When a large proportion of eligible children are vaccinated in a public health program against a human-to-human transmitted pathogen, the disease epidemiology is perturbed – this is called 'herd effect' of vaccination. Herd effect is beneficial to the entire community as the disease frequency is reduced in the vaccinated and unvaccinated segments of population.

For EPI the borders of preventive medicine and public health are blurred. EPI is at once an essential element of primary healthcare as well as a public health program. Eradication is the most ambitious public health program – the entire global population benefits. Polio eradication was incremental additive on to EPI, both benefiting from each other.

Polio eradication could have and should have been achieved through EPI and any obstacles or weaknesses of EPI should have been corrected. After 32 years of polio eradication efforts, is EPI any better than in 1988? Was the mission of eradication hijacked for the purpose of proving that the choice of OPV was the correct choice in EPI? Who other than EPI leaders were actually interested in that idea? The reluctance to use IPV at least in addition to OPV gives away the game. IPV is EPI-compatible and EPI-friendly whereas OPV by campaigns is not, as is well known to all polio workers in all low and middle income countries.

The major problem we face is that polio eradication has not yet been achieved. Benefit delayed is benefit denied. What was promised for 2000 is not yet realized in 2020. Yet, we must not forget that all polio prevented represents benefits both to the individuals and to the community. The problem is regarding the burden of polio that should have been prevented but was not prevented. In other words, the problem is for all those children who have had polio during 2001 through 2020.

For herd effect to be manifested, the vaccine should have high protective efficacy. That is a pre-requisite. High vaccine efficacy and high vaccination coverage may offer sufficient herd effect for interrupting the transmission of the disease agent. That is the basis of disease elimination from large populations, and as applied everywhere, the basis of eradication. It turns out that IPV offers far greater herd effect than OPV, and IPV would have been beneficial to all vaccinated individuals as well as the whole community. If every individual had to be vaccinated against a disease for elimination and eradication, as was the case with OPV, then the goal of elimination/eradication was not attractive – the probability of success would be quite low. This is what happened in all countries that were not able to eliminate wild virus polio by the year 2000 – only because of the exclusive use of OPV that needed to be given to virtually all infants before the age of risk of polio. With a low efficacy vaccine such as OPV, that condition could not be fulfilled – that was why eradication was stalled as long as trivalent OPV was the only OPV available. Eradication of wild viruses became possible only after monovalent types 1 and 3 OPV were licensed and used, since 2005/2006. And, when was the basic scientific information of the 250% higher vaccine efficacy of mOPVs over tOPV available in 1976.[5] Why was that information not applied earlier? Our guess is the unrealistic confidence in tOPV. Hubris, we had mentioned earlier.

India struggled to improve the protective efficacy of OPV (for achieving effectiveness against the circulation of wild polioviruses) with multiple doses of OPV and high immunization coverage. "Failure of vaccine" (consequent to low efficacy) was ignored and the spotlight by the policymakers was on "failure to vaccinate" (a euphemism for falling short of 100%, coverage). Under the polio eradication program the Government pushed hard with multiple OPV campaigns, organized across the country or in selected States, for several years; by 2000 only one wild virus type, type 2, could be eliminated – efficacy of trivalent OPV was about two-and-half times higher for type 2 than for types 1 or 3. In 1999 type 2 wild virus was eliminated; types 1 and 3 wild viruses remained in circulation. Vaccine efficacy of trivalent OPV against wild virus types 1 and 3 were too low to eliminate them in spite of extremely high coverage achieved with it sufficient to eliminate type 2. The lesson is, public health interventions must be designed and applied on the basis of both the ethical principle of benefits and science and not mere belief or assumption.[13]

Compared to benefits of eradication promised by 2000, the reality of polio even in 2020 does not provide pass marks for the ethics principle of benefits for this public health program.

2) Risks

The program should be as safe as possible. The adverse effects should be monitored.

The global polio eradication program cannot be qualified as one with interventions that are 'as safe as possible'. The safety problems have been well described in several chapters in this book. In 2020 OPV-caused polio outnumber natural polio by 600% -- the program does not pass the ethics test of safety – freedom from risk.

In addition to the adverse effects in immunologically normal individuals, OPV harmed children who were immune-deficient (specifically B cell-related immune deficiency), failing the test of the program being 'as safe as possible'. B-cell deficient children had two problems: they had a very high risk of developing VAPP, and they also had a very high risk of developing chronic infection with vaccine viruses.

Such children who became chronically infected with vaccine viruses continued to shed them in their stools for long periods. As they could not mount their own antibody-mediated immunity, they continued to be at risk of polio, and when that happened, the causative virus was back-mutated neurovirulent VDPV, specifically called iVDPV – immune-deficiency associated VDPV.

Chronic infection and continued virus shedding helped the viruses to not only exist in the 'environment' (*i.e.* in infected individuals) but also become more neurovirulent through mutations. This results in polio in the non-immune contacts who themselves were immunologically normal (polio due to infection with iVDPV). The environment has two meanings: poliovirus may survive for weeks in the environment such as sewage, but they cannot survive indefinitely as they gradually die out. Survival of polioviruses in the long term requires infection in human hosts. Now, if I am infected and you are not, for you, I constitute part of your 'environment'.

As for monitoring adverse events, the eradication program was selective in monitoring adverse events. When the most dreaded adverse event, VAPP, occurred in OPV using countries -- that was not monitored. In a public health program initiated after much thought and deliberation, especially backed by highly skilled public health professionals, this omission flies in the face of the public health ethics of safety and the need for monitoring of adverse events.

The other kind of serious adverse events, polio due to community-acquired infection with vaccine-progeny viruses, descendants of the parent vaccine viruses, in other words VDPVs, could not be ignored or swept under the carpet. As infection is community-acquired, the virus is already in outbreak mode and circulating; ignoring it would be at the peril of the program itself. So VDPVs were carefully monitored. Such monitoring required 'environmental surveillance' – a term applied to the monitoring of sewage samples for the presence of VDPV – so that the outbreak of infection could be detected even before cases occur – or the extent of the outbreak of infection could be ascertained. Thus, environmental surveillance fulfilled partly the principle of monitoring adverse events, but it exposed the inconvenient truth of the magnitude of the problem. There were 183 and 196 VDPV isolations from healthy children in contact with paralysed children in 2019 and 2020, respectively. There were also 224 and 352 VDPV isolations from sewage samples in various countries, in 2019 and 2020 respectively.

The eradication program relying solely on OPV does not satisfy the qualification: 'as safe as possible', as the complete safety of IPV was deliberately avoided, thus vitiating the ethical principle under discussion. The problem of paralytic polio caused by OPV became more evident with time, as numbers of VAPP apparently rose in countries using OPV, as the OPV coverage increased. VAPP was counted in India only two decades after the introduction of OPV, despite the early advice by WHO to monitor adverse events (VAPP) after implementing the EPI with OPV. VAPP numbers were 181, 129 and 109 in the years 1999, 2000 and 2001 respectively.[2] The highest number of VAPP occurred in children 1–4 years of age. The majority affected were children who had received more than three doses of OPV prior to onset.

In the USA, after the introduction of OPV, VAPP cases increased from 12 in the year 1965 to 16 in 1972. USA has had the best data on VAPP. What about European countries? In 1976, an enquiry started earlier by WHO, into the relationship between OPV and VAPP, was published; it confirmed VAPP in all European countries using OPV.[14] Despite VAPP, the report asserted, strangely, that OPV was 'one of the safest vaccines in use.'[15]

Subsequent follow-up publications related to this enquiry by the WHO was in 1982 and 1988; they also repeatedly asserted that "OPV was one of the safest vaccines in use" despite the global reports of VAPP cases caused by OPV.[16,17] Albert Sabin, the scientist who developed Sabin OPV was also a member of the enquiry committee; he clearly had a conflict of interest, and the committee's disinterestedness or even-handedness – lack of bias in other words -- was compromised.[17]

WHO, as world leader in the art and science of public health, has, for decades, maintained a Committee on Vaccine Safety, which scrutinises all issues regarding the safety of all vaccines. In May 2014 the Committee put out an information sheet on vaccine reactions of OPV and IPV. [18] IPV was reported not to cause any serious adverse events. OPV, on the other hand, was reported to cause the following serious adverse reactions: Vaccine associated paralytic polio, VAPP; Vaccine-derived polioviruses causing polio; Aseptic meningitis/Encephalitis in immunodeficient infants. We are not aware if the polio eradication program took note of this information and if it it did, how it justified the continued use of OPV without pre-protection using IPV against serious adverse reactions to OPV.

By 2000, USA discontinued use of OPV and adopted the policy of exclusive use of IPV. While many developed countries shifted to IPV, WHO continued to promote the use of OPV in developing countries. By another decade, as all high-income countries switched to IPV, over 90% of the VAPP burden got geographically confined to low- and low-middle-income countries which had continued the exclusively use of OPV.[17]

As the information on paralysis caused by vaccine viruses mounted, the eradication program came up with another strategy in 1995. This strategy was adopted in the first Consultative meeting of the Global Commission for Certification (GCC) of Poliomyelitis held in Geneva in 1995. The GCC defined global polio eradication as "the eradication of all wild polioviruses", and specified that "the occurrence of clinical cases of poliomyelitis caused by other enteroviruses, **including attenuated polio vaccine viruses,** does not invalidate the achievement of wild poliovirus eradication."[19]

Knowing very well that polio eradication can be realized only in the absence of cVDPV, the SAGE Polio Working Group Committee requested the WHO to develop a separate process for verifying the absence of cVDPV in the 'post-certification era', after 'cessation of oral poliovirus vaccine use.'[20]

The experts obviously believed that after eradication of wild polioviruses using OPV, OPV could be withdrawn when all vaccine-related polio would disappear – VAPP for sure should disappear, but what about cVDPVs? As we stated in the chapter on Proof of Principle and Country Models (Chapter 7), there was no precedent of 'cessation of OPV' in the absence of high coverage IPV in any country. Why would the eradication program avoid time tested principle but use an untested modality?

This strange attitude of the policymakers of the program could be best explained as "normalisation of deviance". The term means that people within the organisation become so much accustomed to a deviant behaviour that they don't consider it as deviant, despite the fact that they far exceed their own rules for the elementary safety."

This concept and its name were described by an American Sociologist, Diane Vaughan, who attributed it as a cause for a dangerous flaw in the design and testing of the NASA spaceship shuttle "The Challenger."[21] NASA officials continued to permit space shuttle missions despite evidence of a design flaw in the solid rocket boosters. Instead of objectively evaluating the risks, the unacceptable standards were gradually passed on by the officials as acceptable because inaction on their part had not caused any negative consequence. The repeated deviant behaviour by the officials became a sort of a 'social norm' in NASA and ultimately became responsible for the catastrophic failure of the Challenger on 28th January 1986, killing seven astronauts who were on board.

Despite the scientific evidence emerging from India (and many other low-income countries) about the poor seroconversion rates following OPV, the known adverse effects of VAPP and polio due to VDPVs, and excellent efficacy of the completely safe IPV, those involved in the global polio eradication program overlooked the crucial flaw in the choice of vaccine and repeatedly asserted the safety of the unsafe OPV vaccine in its official declarations.

People working outside the organization who might not have been involved in the cultural drift of accepting the unacceptable could have looked at the flaw with an unblinded eye and recognized the flaw as unacceptable. Again this did not happen in case of the policymakers in India for example who also shared the attitude of "normalization of deviance" manifested by the decision-makers of the program. Possibly the policymakers of India were heavily influenced by the program experts who might have convinced them that they are also 'insiders' in the global program.

Papua New Guinea had a polio outbreak due to cVDPV type 1 in 2018 after remaining free from natural polio for about 18 years.[22] Similarly, Syria also had an outbreak due to cVDPV type 2 in 2017 after remaining without a single case of natural polio for two decades.[23] Both these countries had observed more polio than countries like Pakistan and Afghanistan which have not yet achieved polio-free status till date due to various problems related to community resistance to OPV vaccine campaigns and internal conflicts.

In December 2020, Sierra Leone in West Africa, detected 3 children with polio paralysis after ten years of absence of any polio. The virus has been confirmed as cVDPV type 2.[24] Large outbreaks of polio due to cVDPV -2 were reported in 2020 in Chad, DR Congo, Sudan, Cote d'Ivoire, Burkina Faso, Pakistan and Afghanistan.

The test of risks under public health ethics does not show that the program passed it.

3) Effectiveness

The program should be effective and should not be allowed to continue if not effective.

Effectiveness is producing the intended result. But the program has failed so far to achieve its target.

Using a mathematical calculation based on the data of VAPP available from CDC, we constructed a graph (Fig 8.1) which represents the total number of polio cases, namely cases of VAPP plus polio cases due to VDPVs resulting from the continued OPV based program.[25]

The annual VAPP cases in India were 100-200 prior to 2016 when the trivalent OPV was switched to bivalent OPV.[26] In other words; there was an average of 150 cases per year i.e. 12 per month before 2016. Let us now look at the effect of the global switch from trivalent to bivalent OPV and simultaneous introduction of IPV. The exclusive use of trivalent OPV vaccine leads to VAPP due to type 2 vaccine virus in 26% recipients (recipient VAPP) and 31% contacts (contact VAPP). Therefore type 2 withdrawal would lead to a reduction in VAPP by at least 25 to 30%. Since IPV protects against VAPP, it was predicted that the withdrawal of type 2 from OPV with the simultaneous introduction of IPV could reduce the overall VAPP cases by up to 90%.[27]

However, due to delay in acquiring IPV for use in national immunization schedule due to a global shortage of the vaccine, we have assumed at least 50% reduction.[28] Since the switch took place in April 2016, we have counted 12 per month till April and 6 for the remaining 8 months. Since India's population is about 1/5th the population of developing countries,[29]we have multiplied the Indian data by 5 to obtain the global data of VAPP, i.e. 750 cases till 2015, 480 in 2016 and 360 post OPV switch.

CDC data also gives a count of cases of Immune-deficiency associated VDPV (iVDPV) and Ambiguous VDPV (aVDPV) periodically with some reports having an overlap of 3-6 months. Using the average per month calculated from each report and multiplied with 12, data provides us with 5 cases of iVDPV cases and 10 cases of aVDPV cases per year.[30-33]

The graph, drawn based on this arithmetic calculation, reveals the shocking picture of the large numbers of polio cases that the program continues to cause, far more than natural polio due to wild polioviruses.[34-38]

As illustrated in the graph, of the total polio cases in 2008, two-thirds were due to wild polioviruses, and one third was due to vaccine viruses. The benefit-risk ratio of the vaccine used in the program is clearly unacceptable. Also, if the polio cases due to vaccine viruses had occurred in countries free of wild polioviruses, there benefit-risk ratio fell in the negative zone, less than zero. Despite the negative benefit value, the program continued using OPV exclusively until 2015.

Children who developed program-induced polio all the years since 2000, were not the same children in whom wild viruses would have caused polio.

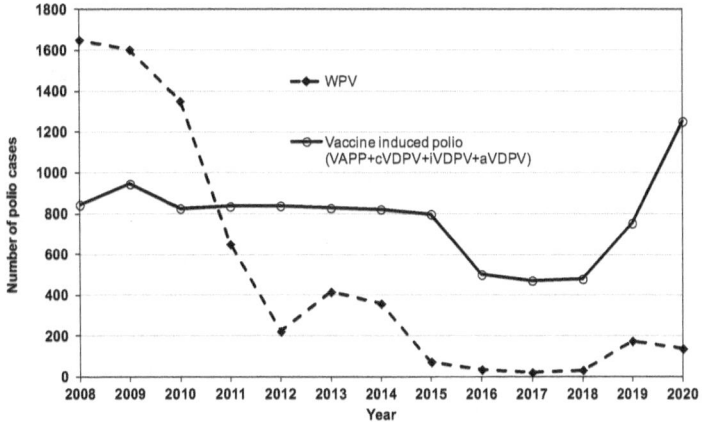

Fig 8.1: *Annual numbers of polio due to Wild Polio Viruses (WPV) and estimated numbers of polio due to vaccine and vaccine-lineage polioviruses (VAPP, cVDPV, iVDPV and aVDPV). The vaccine-induced VAPP is neither monitored nor counted. Among the vaccine-lineage cases, cVDPV (circulating vaccine derived polio virus) cases are monitored and counted. Polio caused by iVDPV (Immune-deficiency associated VDPV) and aVDPV (Ambiguous VDPV) are not counted regularly. Therefore, we have extrapolated their annual numbers from the available data.*

No public health program has the right to shift risks from one to another or one group to another group.

Clearly, the ethical principle of effectiveness is not fulfilled and the program is not effective enough to be continued in the present form -- if the program takes public health ethics seriously. A course correction is the need of the hour. Course correction had been long overdue.

4) Equity and justice

The program should be cost-effective. Priority should be provided to the most vulnerable population.

a. The program should be cost-effective

Cost-effectiveness studies had concluded that the eradication program as such was theoretically cost effective.[36,37] The first study was in 1996, anticipating rapid eradication within a few years; hence its conclusion is no longer valid. The second study was conducted in 2010, and now we are in 2020 – so, the conclusions are not to be taken at its face value.

Low-income countries were estimated to account for 85% incremental net benefits (approximately 40-50 billion dollars) of the program between 1988 and 2035, despite the high costs of the program in these countries.[39]

None of these studies has evaluated the ethics of the use of OPV to the exclusion of IPV. OPV requires almost 100 per cent coverage with repeated doses whereas 85-90% coverage with 2-3 doses of IPV should be sufficient to prevent polio due to wild or vaccine viruses – in other words, 2-3 IPV doses have much higher efficacy than multiple doses of OPV and on account of the very high vaccine efficacy we could expect higher herd effect than with OPV at any coverage level.

A cost-effectiveness study supporting eradication program included 392 reported cases with VDPV between 2000 and 2009 in 104 countries – for an annual average of about 39 cases, but in 2018 itself there were 104 cases in 8 countries.[40] The number of cases has more than tripled in 2019 with ~388 cases of VDPV. Therefore the problems caused by the use of OPV were grossly underestimated by the economists. Vaccination campaigns cost approximately US $ one billion per year. According to a 2015 midterm review by the Bill and Melinda Gates Foundation, (an important donor agency for the program), an additional US $ 1.5 billion was required to fund the program through 2019.[40] In the current scenario of VDPV outbreaks occurring in 25 countries, and the failure to eradicate wild polioviruses for over three decades, it is high time that the donor agencies question the failing strategies of the current program and the grossly misleading economic predictions. We suspect that the OPV-centric polio eradication program may not be as cost-effective as an all-IPV eradication program.

b. Priority should be provided to the most vulnerable population.

The dictionary meaning of vulnerability is, "the quality or state of being exposed to the possibility of being attacked or harmed, either physically or emotionally."[41] Vulnerable population in health care context include children, elderly, socioeconomically disadvantaged, under-insured, those with certain medical conditions or those who belong to racial or ethnic minority populations.[42]

These groups are at risk of inadequate access to care and therefore, tend to suffer the worst health outcome. Children in low and middle-income countries do not have access to complete rehabilitation or monetary compensation if affected by polio due to vaccine virus. The polio victims not only face physical and emotional suffering but also significant social barriers which push them to further poverty. Children of these countries must be classified as a vulnerable population for the global polio eradication program. Therefore the program has an obligation to offer topmost priority to this group and provide them IPV, which is devoid of serious adverse effects that OPV cause in them and will also protect them from polio due to vaccine viruses.

5) Autonomy

Sufficient information about the risks and benefits should be provided to the vaccine recipients or parents of the children to be able to make an autonomous decision. There should not be any kind of force applied for participation.

By policy of one vaccine (OPV), autonomy for member nations and professional bodies in countries, and to parents was denied. The program was not transparent in informing the risks associated with OPV-- VAPP and VDPV, to the communities and countries..

There was little public communication that a live vaccine was used, and those with immune deficiency or their siblings should not take the vaccine to prevent the increased risk of VAPP. People and countries were also kept in the dark about the reason that required it to be administered multiple times till 5 years of age – namely, it's very poor efficacy per dose. The repetitive vaccine inoculation, particularly making sure that girl children were not missed, was one reason why antipathy to OPV developed in some communities in Nigeria, Pakistan and Afghanistan. In our assessment the ethical principle of autonomy was severely compromised by the programme while insisting on the exclusive use of OPV.

6) Reciprocity

Medical care should be provided to those who suffer from any serious adverse event due to vaccination. Also no-fault compensation should be given to the victims.

The USA had made provisions for compensation of those who suffered adverse effects of the polio vaccine under the National Childhood Vaccine Injury Act of 1986. Although the first compensation under this Act was awarded in 1988, lawsuits against vaccine manufacturers had hit the national headlines since the 1970s. For instance, in May 1970, when 8-month-old Anita Reyes was diagnosed with paralytic poliomyelitis after two weeks of receiving trivalent oral polio vaccine manufactured by Wyeth, the jury in the USA gave a verdict in favour of Reyes family a sum of $200,000 on the grounds of improper warning to the family about the risk of developing polio from the vaccine prior to administering it to

Anita.[43] As many more similar claims for vaccines were filed, some manufacturers began to lose interest in not so lucrative business and withdrew from vaccine production. To ensure a continued interest by the vaccine manufacturers and stability in vaccine supply, the US Congress passed the National Childhood Vaccine Injury Act of 1986. Through this Act the Government became responsible "to compensate the children who have been injured while serving the public good." Vaccine companies had to increase vaccine price in order to make profit in spite of litigation. As lawsuits for VAPP cases had increased across the country, the US Government started worrying about the safety of oral polio vaccine and its adverse effects on the country's reputation, and as 2000 was the target year for polio eradication, USA finally abandoned OPV altogether in 2000. Thus USA passed the reciprocity clause of ethics in 2000.

Several countries in Europe have similarly established a no-fault compensation scheme. Ethics related to a public health program cannot change based on whether the program is being delivered to a developing or a developed country, or whether the national Government or a global agency is responsible for its delivery. Polio, whether VAPP or due to VDPV, is a serious adverse event of the vaccine. As per the principle of reciprocity, rehabilitation services should have been proved free of cost and monetary compensation provided for the disability caused. However, children with VAPP were not even identified by the program, let alone compensated. The same fate has been met with children who became victims of VDPV outbreaks. In other words, the ethical principle of reciprocity is simply nonexistent as far as the eradication program is concerned.

7) Trust

It is important to preserve public trust in the program . Participation should be encouraged through discussions in a

public forum like meetings, etc.

Public trust in the program is of paramount importance. Vaccine hesitancy was identified in 2019 as one of the ten top global threats. The Strategic Advisory Group of Experts (SAGE) Working Group on Vaccine Hesitancy described vaccine hesitancy as delay in acceptance or refusal, of vaccination, despite the availability of vaccination services.[44]

Loss of trust in vaccination program may occur due to religious or philosophical beliefs or due to fear about the safety of the vaccine as discussed below: Open communication and transparency could help minimize vaccine hesitancy. Concerns were raised by the Independent Monitoring Board on Polio Eradication that, "*Within the Program, communications is the poor cousin of vaccine delivery, undeservedly receiving far less focus. Communications expertise is sparse throughout and needs to be strengthened.*"[44]

Since 2012, at least 100 polio workers have been killed in Pakistan. Recently in April 2019 in Pakistan, a polio worker and two policemen escorting the vaccination teams were shot dead by militants. Pakistan was forced to suspend the vaccination campaign at a time when polio due to wild polioviruses was on the rise. Pakistan is now at high risk for outbreaks of both WPV-1 and by cVDPVs, as the vaccine viruses spread to the unvaccinated children and back-mutate. Since OPV is given multiple times, there is a perception in the community that it has a hidden purpose of reducing fertility. In such a situation, IPV vaccines administered with the routine EPI vaccines can escape the attention of militants who have targeted the OPV immunization program.[45]

Vaccine hesitancy can be best mitigated with community participation, transparency and education about the benefits and risks. In the era of growing vaccine hesitancy, the program should now formulate corrective measures to implement policies that will best reduce the risks resulting due to vaccine hesitancy.

We doubt if trust can be regained in many communities and countries as long as the program insists of giving repeated doses of OPV, not in response to the occurrence of polio but to pre-empt the occurrence of polio due to the very same vaccine that is promoted to prevent polio due to it. The program is losing grip on reality in so many countries that continue to have polio paralysis that the program celebrates as not polio due to natural viruses. That distinction may satisfy the program personnel – but for the paralysed children and their families that information is of no comfort whatsoever. Children are paralysed for their entire life time.

Summation

The use of OPV in the eradication program beyond 2000 has been increasingly associated with more harm than benefit. If drugs and vaccines have been withdrawn by regulatory bodies when they failed to perform their utility, or if the basic ethical principles of beneficence and non-maleficence are not fulfilled, OPV should also meet the same fate on ethical grounds. In routine immunisation in primary healthcare or in EPI, the use of OPV has serious ethical problems. A valid ethics assessment does not show OPV to be an ethical choice as long as the safe alternate vaccine IPV is available,

Moreover, the current program does not appear to meet the principles public health ethics. Every one of the seven ethics principles of immunisation program under public health -- Benefits, Risks, Effectiveness, Equity and justice, Autonomy, Reciprocity and Trust, is not satisfied by the program. In the current era of vaccine hesitancy, the program must ensure that public trust is created and maintained by transparency and effective communication. Alternate truth, like stating that "OPV is one of the safest vaccines" cannot alter truth. If transparency is compromised on one vaccine, it may affect other vaccines too.

We echo Skrabanek's observation that medical interventions (read immunisation), even when applied in the name of preventive medicine or health promotion, do not absolve the program promoters of adherence in letter and spirit, to the prescriptions of healthcare ethics and public health ethics. The mere good intention to eradicate polio does not justify the program from veering out of the perimeter drawn by ethics. .

With program-induced polio outbreaks in 19 countries in 2019, and 25 countries in 2020, it may be likened to running a recklessly driven vehicle, without a clear destination in sight. Drastic corrective measures have become the need of the hour. What is the destination and what is the roadmap? The next chapter explains the lack of focus on the destination. Now the program is wandering in the wilderness.

§§§

9. WANDERING IN WILDERNESS

Sandipthe bhavane tu koopa khananam prati udyama ki
drusya? (Sanskrit: What do you think of someone digging a well
when the house is on fire?)

Polio eradication can be likened to a journey with its starting
point (Point A), a checkpoint (Point B) and the final
destination (Point C). The checkpoint *en route* is to give
confidence that the path from A to C is correct and progress
satisfactory. The Journey began in 1988. The intention was to
reach Point C by 2000. We are now in 2020, and have not yet
crossed Point B; when do you think we can reach Point C?

The story so far: the inconvenient scientific information

The eradication journey began in 1988. The viruses to be
eradicated were wild poliovirus (WPV) types 1, 2 and 3.
Eradication had to be achieved without allowing the live
viruses in the Sabin OPV, also types 1, 2 and 3, gaining a
foothold in the community as endemic (spreading from the
infected to the uninfected). Great caution was called for,

since in 1988 the majority of countries in the world were vaccinating children with OPV under the Expanded Program on Immunisation (EPI).

The vaccine viruses were not completely attenuated, but retained very low neurovirulence, causing vaccine-associated paralytic polio (VAPP) and very low transmissibility, causing occasional horizontal child to child spread of infection. Another risk with the use of OPV was the propensity of the vaccine virus strains to drift towards the genetic makeup of the parental wild polioviruses.

The drift back to virulence starts with the multiplication of the Sabin-original (SO) virus in cell culture, each generation numbered starting with 1 -- as SO+1, and progressively increasing through SO+2 and SO+3 and so on. The virus in the OPV vials are usually in the spectrum of minimum SO+4 but maximum unknown, which could be between SO+5 and SO+10 or even more. What is the importance of knowing these minutiae of manufacturing details? Known only to virologists, not informed to the public, is the fact that every dose of OPV, even at SO+4, in the vial, contains a minute number of genetically back-drifted neurovirulent viruses diluted among the vast majority of non-drifted SO-like viruses.[1,2] More number of generations would mean more back-drifted viruses. The consequence of this reality is VAPP in vaccinated children. That is unavoidable. If we must predictably protect against VAPP, we must vaccinate first with at least one dose of IPV and then only give OPV.

This idea of giving at least one dose of IPV at 14 weeks of age was used in 2016 as formal recommendation by the polio eradication program and WHO, prior to withdrawing type 2 from trivalent OPV. The globally synchronous switch from trivalent OPV (tOPV) to bivalent OPV (bOPV) was achieved in April 2016. That "at least one dose of IPV" step was qualified as "risk mitigation" strategy. What risk was there to mitigate when one type virus was actually being removed from OPV? That begs the questions why remove type 2 virus and what risk its removal would pose? Commonsense would suggest that removing a virus from inoculation should remove any risk: here it is, oddly, the opposite. Removing posed a risk.

2000 came and went with no success. Every subsequent target set by the program was missed. Now after 16 years of wandering without seeing even a glimpse of El Dorado, the program had to be extremely careful in making no more false moves.

The risk of VAPP in the vaccinated was more with type 3 Sabin virus than with types 2 or 1. The risk of VAPP in contact children was more with type 2 than with types 3 or 1. This was widely known among all polio experts and virologists right from the 1970s and 1980s. These findings had been documented by the WHO Committee on Polio vaccines and published in the Bulletins of WHO. Now for one inconvenient information: the type 2 virus in the vaccine vial is less transmissible and less neurovirulent than the type 2 virus in a child infected with vaccine virus, as it would have multiplied through many more generations.

What kept type 2 vaccine virus from becoming endemic (meaning transmitting from children to children in the community) until 2006, was the background community immunity derived from wild type 2 virus that had circulated widely during the 1990s and was eradicated in 1999. From 2006, after a grace period of 6 years since 1999, circulating vaccine-derived poliovirus type 2 (VDPV-2) began causing polio outbreaks in Nigeria. The grace period was missed by the program – in spite of specific request to that effect.[3]

High community immunity had to be achieved by the repeated feeding of all children (or as many as possible) with tOPV from the vials, in order to stem the tide that began in 2006. OPV feeding was necessary to prevent vaccine virus type 2 from becoming more of a menace in the community.

However, more OPV resulted also in more opportunities for type 2 to emerge as cVDPV. Finally, wisdom dawned and it was decided to remove type 2 from tOPV in 2016, seventeen years after wild type 2 was eradicated and when the only polio paralysis caused by type 2 virus was by vaccine virus type 2. Principles of ethics and epidemiology were not followed. Since April 2016 only bivalent OPV (bOPV) containing types 1 and 3 is routinely given in the program.

Removing type 2 from immunizing children posed the risk of vaccine-derived type 2 virus from becoming endemic and causing VAPP in the community. Full immunizing schedule of two IPV doses would have ensured full protection from both community-acquired VAPP due to type 2 and from sustained community transmission of type 2. The program gambled on deciding on only one dose. The hope was that one dose of IPV would be sufficient to prevent Sabin type 2 virus already in the children who had been vaccinated up to the date of the tOPV to bOPV switch, from further transmission. Unfortunately, the plan failed: vaccine-derived type 2 virus emerged in too many communities and caused polio in several non-immune children and also spread widely and even got exported to other countries.

The intention of one dose IPV was "risk mitigation", not protection from contact VAPP. Two doses of IPV would have protected children from polio whether caused by WPV or vaccine virus from the vial or vaccine lineage virus from other children. Two doses would have expedited global polio eradication also.

But that was not to be. There was some tight rope walking here. The extreme reluctance on the part of the program to use any IPV at all, from the beginning of the program, was widely known. Suddenly, if the program relaxed its tight grip on IPV, and recommended two doses, the message would have been that IPV was superior to OPV as it would protect from VAPP and cVDPV; hence it was also effective against

WPV. That would be, rather could have been, the beginning of the end of (1) the dependence of the program solely on OPV; (2) the eradication program itself as all polio would be prevented; (3) the faith in the program's dogma of the need for OPV and avoidance of IPV.

The program had to be very careful. But it was not – there is a saying that things do go wrong if you give them a chance. Deep scientific knowledge, conviction for being ethical, sense of accountability to the donors and to the people being served, wisdom not to take avoidable risks – all these were necessary to veer the program through the wilderness that it was sixteen years after the missed target, back on track. Let us begin at the beginning.

Planning for the journey

How do we describe Point A? It is not a geographic location but a global situation that existed at the starting point, 1988. Similarly, the destination (Point C) too – can be defined as a global situation that will meet all demands of a 'totally polio-free world'.

Totally polio-free means that there should be no natural source of poliovirus infection anywhere in the world and all polio vaccination could be (theoretically) stopped without fear or risk of infection from natural sources. If poliovirus survived in any person, that would be a natural source of infection – therefore, by definition, no one should be infected – hence no natural source of infection in any community anywhere in the world. The absence of extra-human reservoir as a source of poliovirus was one of the reasons why polio was targeted for eradication. This much was learned from the one and only eradication precedent in human diseases, that of smallpox eradication. In the animal world, rinderpest also has been eradicated with rinderpest vaccine.

The world had changed much and in many ways from the time of smallpox eradication to the time of starting the polio eradication journey. Therefore, some new potential risks had to be imagined. Wild polioviruses could be, would be, kept viable in too many virus laboratories in too many countries to be counted with comfort and confidence that they will not become a source. When smallpox was eradicated there were only very few virus laboratories working on smallpox virus – they could be counted on the fingers of one hand. In the case of poliovirus, innumerable labs in many countries had worked with polioviruses. Any laboratory leak of wild poliovirus would be a potential risk. The vaccine polioviruses, due to their tendency for transmission and genetic reversion by mutations, are in the same league with wild polioviruses as far as potential risks are concerned, in a polio-eradicated world.

Stool samples, nose swabs and throat swabs that had been collected for various purposes, not only for poliovirus work but also for work on viruses of the respiratory and gastrointestinal tracts, and held in deep freezers, would also be a possible source of polioviruses. Clinical specimens collected for bacteriology would not usually be stored in deep freezers.

A virus could accidentally leak from storage in virus laboratories and pose a risk – any infection in any person, adults included, could spread rapidly as the community will have many non-immune children unless vaccination coverage is kept high. So, although the risk of infection from a natural source would be zero, risk of infection from a virus in laboratory storage had to be considered, for which reason, polio vaccination should not be stopped in a hurry even after reaching Point C. That much should have been, indeed it was, very obvious to the polio eradication program experts at Point A itself.

The global polio eradication program has an elaborate plan, protocol and standard operating procedures to mitigate such risks. The serially revised versions of global action plans for poliovirus containment, wild as well as vaccine, are to be highly appreciated. Let us go back to the time of pre-Point A when the journey was being planned.

When imagining the destination, Point C, the following would have been clear. Any polio vaccination at and after Point C, had to be obviously with only IPV. In other words, OPV will be incompatible for use as it contains infectious polioviruses, albeit attenuated. Vaccine polioviruses are transmissible (as they are incompletely attenuated) and their attenuation is reversible (another sign of incomplete attenuation) -- and these are important reasons why OPV had to be prohibited before we could reach Point C.

Since vaccine viruses could remain in vaccinated children or their contacts in their families and peer groups, for some weeks, even months, OPV should be stopped from use for a fairly long period of time before the world would reach Point C.

Let us designate as Point B, the checkpoint, as the point in time beyond which no OPV should be in use. So the polio eradication journey is from Point A (1988, when both IPV and OPV were in use in different countries) to Point B (when any use of OPV anywhere should be stopped) and from Point B to Point C (during which period of time only IPV should be used). The path from Point B to Point C is necessary to ensure that all vaccine-lineage viruses die out in the community, or are interrupted deliberately using IPV. Needless to say WPV should have been interrupted from transmission in all erstwhile OPV-using countries that had WPV in circulation – either before or after reaching point B.

Points A and C were clarified as global situations with categorical characteristics. Point B is a global situation that needed clarification.

What is Point B?

Simply put, Point B is that global situation wherein all use of OPV could be discontinued and only IPV is in use. All along in this book, in several chapters, we had been highlighting this crucial message – that OPV should have been discontinued (at Point B) ideally well ahead of the target year 2000 (the original set-point for Point C), or at least by 2000 (having realized that the journey was not on the right road map), or latest as soon after 2000 as possible (when the world had a crisis on hand with polio eradication target missed by a wide margin). Polio eradication had lost its way by 2000 and has not yet come back on the real route which has to touch the checkpoint Point B to know that the route is correct.

When could all use of OPV be safely discontinued? Well, that was something that should have been part of the planning of the journey of polio eradication. The issue was not based on science alone – it was also based on practical considerations. In 1988 all low and middle-income countries were using OPV exclusively. Point B demanded that all countries switch to IPV and to the exclusive use of IPV. Thereafter polio surveillance would have shown where any poliovirus (WPV or vaccine poliovirus) was circulating. There IPV use had to be intensified so that each line of virus transmission, irrespective of wild or vaccine, was broken – for reaching Point C. So, the timing of discontinuation was a choice for the program to make, in 1988 itself. A simple approach would have been half the time, six years, for the journey from Point A to Point B and six years from Point B to Point C -- that is, assuming that the program had clearly understood the issues involved. What seems to us is that the program had not understood the issues involved. That is illustrated in Fig 9.1A as the roadmap the program had originally designed and had to modify later.

The program's original plan was to use OPV exclusively to reach the point when all wild polioviruses were eradicated under OPV and then to allow countries a choice either to discontinue OPV to avoid any VAPP or continue OPV living with some VAPP. Then the problem of cVDPV 2 outbreaks started in 2006. The original plan of exclusive use of OPV had to be modified in 2016, and one dose of IPV was introduced. The journey was to continue towards a world without wild virus polio and cVDPV-2 polio. But, even after removing type 2 from OPV in 2016, the risk of further emergence of cVDPV-2 could not be mitigated, but further emergence continued to happen with increased prevalence in more geographic communities and increased frequency.

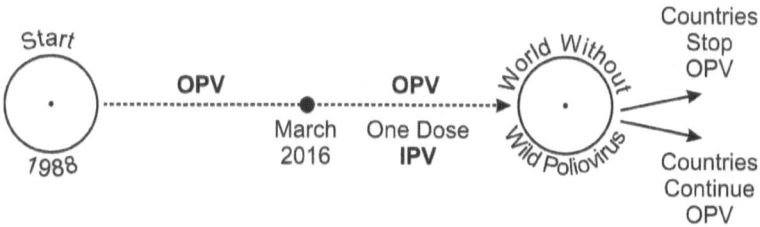

Fig 9.1A: *Cartoon depicting the path designed by the polio eradication program. The starting point was 1988; destination was defined as a world without wild poliovirus, accepting vaccine virus polio as adverse reaction to OPV. There was no plan to eradicate vaccine viruses. After reaching zero wild virus status, countries were to decide to continue or discontinue OPV. IPV had no role assigned. Since March 2016, every child is to be given one dose of IPV at or after 14 weeks of age, as explained in the text.*

This conundrum of how the program is wandering in the wilderness is depicted in Fig 9.1 B. The program is wandering between Point A and Point B but there is no indication that the journey is looking for Point B. In other words, the program is now become a vaccine delivery platform, plus a superb polio and poliovirus surveillance program. The significance of the destinations of Point B and thereafter Point C seems not to have been understood at all.

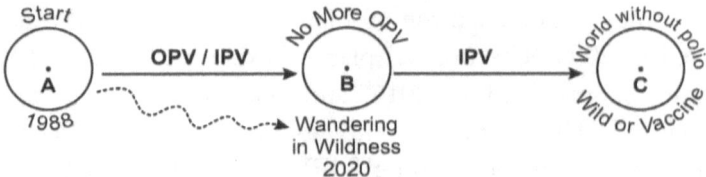

Fig 9.1B: *Cartoon depicting the path the polio eradication program should have adopted. The destination (Point C) should have been a world without polio, any polio -- wild virus caused or vaccine virus caused. Only IPV should have been in use and any vaccine virus in community circulation should have died out or stopped with IPV. Between Point A and Point B, IPV should have been introduced and ramped up and OPV ramped down until Point B when all OPV should have been stopped.*

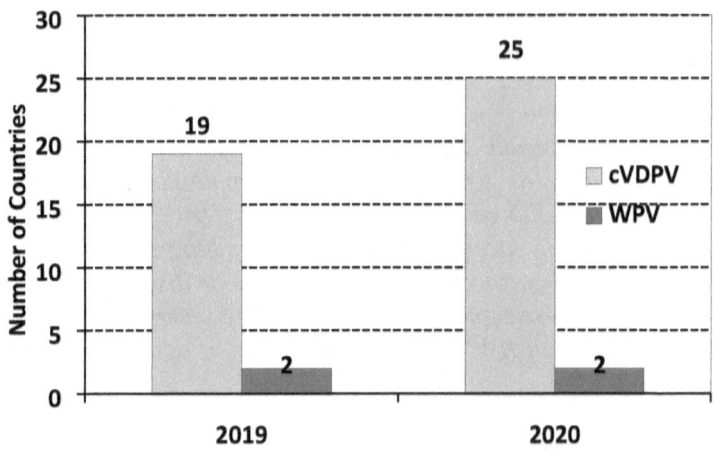

Fig 9.2A: *Number of countries that reported polio due to circulating vaccine-derived polio viruses (cVDPV) and polio due to wild polio virus (WPV), in the years 2019 and 2020 (data up to 23 December 2020)*

In 2019 and 2020 polio outbreaks due to circulating de-attenuated vaccine viruses had been recorded in 19 and 25 countries, respectively (see Figure 9.2 A). The need for protecting all children in all low income countries from vaccine-induced polio by at least two doses of IPV in EPI is urgent, but the market is now IPV sellers' market. In 1988, as the enhanced potency IPV was popular and not highly expensive, it would have been fairly easy to get as much IPV as the world needed, if only the program policy did not exclude IPV. Then it was a buyers' market.

Since IPV was excluded from the program the message was loud and clear to the vaccine industry – there would be no demand for high volume for maintaining low price. Demand remained high in rich countries, in which the requirement was relatively small, and market forces led to low-volume-high-price spiral. Today if the program wants to reach Point B quickly, the needed IPV may not be available in the market and what is available would be unaffordable to the program. Double damage has befallen the program.

The consequences of wandering

When the program started in 1988 there were three serotypes of wild polioviruses in many OPV-using countries to be eradicated. One serotype, type 2, was eradicated in 1999. Instead of discontinuing the type 2 component in OPV, it was continued in a world in which the background high herd immunity to wild type 2 was declining. Eventually, type 2 vaccine viruses began evolving into vaccine derived neurovirulent viruses that were also regaining transmission efficiency. This tactical error, not taking the right steps at the right time, has been a recurrent feature of the program -- that was because of not defining Point B.

In 2012 type 3 wild virus was eradicated, but vaccine virus type 3 is still in wide use, causing some VAPP that remains hidden as they are not counted. There is no epidemiological need for type 3 OPV anymore, since 2016. Fortunately type 3 is less prone to become circulating VDPV. Still, why take a chance of letting type 3 vaccine virus having free run for genetic reversion to virulence? Now the program faces only type 1 wild virus for eradication, and that too in just two countries. Do we need type 1 OPV in countries that have had no WPV 1 for decades?

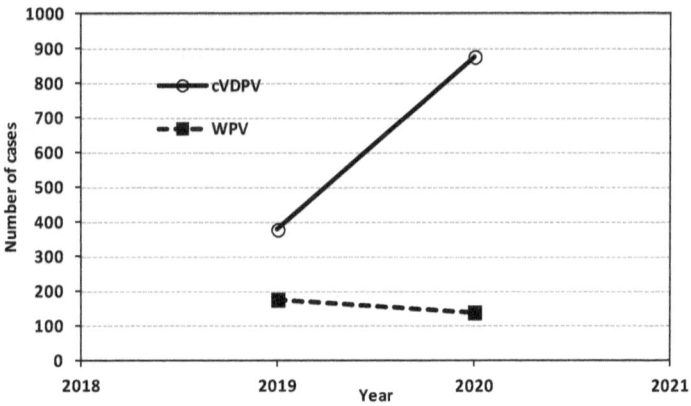

Fig 9.2B: *Number of polio cases caused by Circulating Vaccine-derived Polio viruses (cVDPV) and Wild Polio Virus (WPV), in the years 2019 (378 cVDPV and 176 WPV) and 2020 (876 cVDPV and 139 WPV). VAPP and polio caused by other vaccine-lineage viruses (iVDPV and aVDPV) are not included in the graph. The total number of polio caused by the vaccine viruses in 2020 will exceed 1200 if they are also added to the number of cVDPV cases.*

However, cVDPV-2 polio is occurring in 25 countries as of now. Now the program has to eradicate it also from the world. Had the program planned to reach Point B, the journey towards the completion of eradication would have been rather straightforward.

Eradication program should have ensured that vaccine viruses did not circulate, regain neurovirulence and become a second and sinister target agent for eradication. Now, in 2020, the vaccine-lineage viruses are affecting twelve times as many countries than those affected by natural polio (Fig 9.2 A) and causing six times more polio cases than natural polioviruses (See Fig 9.2 B). The vaccine-lineage viruses are more difficult to eradicate than natural polioviruses if we keep on using OPV. If IPV is given to all children, vaccine-polio can be prevented and then it will be far easier to eradicate both wild and vaccine viruses together.

A goal without timeline, a journey without destination

Point A is behind us, 32 years ago. We have not reached Point C. Is Point C at least visible in the distance? You cannot look out for Point C without reaching point B. As long as we use OPV in any country, we have not yet reached Point B. The program has lost its way and is wandering in the wilderness (Fig 9.1 B). It has lost its way between Point A and Point B. We have to reach point B first, and then only we can travel to Point C.

So, it was very important to have described and defined Point B – that global situation when we could have safely discontinued all OPV from all countries. In 2020, the program still has its staple as OPV. The world cannot reach Point C before first reaching point B.

The error that the program seems to have made was, not defining Points B and C. The program drew a mental map – Point A to C without considering Point B. (Fig 9.1 A). The destination, Point C was erroneously defined by the program as a world without wild polioviruses and not a world without any poliovirus in circulation, wild and vaccine.

The correct route ought to have been Point A to B to C (Fig 9.1 B). We repeat: the program leadership had imagined that wild polioviruses should be eradicated first, for which OPV was selected exclusively as the tool, and then to let countries decide whether to continue OPV or discontinue OPV. They did not comprehend that the true polio-free world, Point C as we describe, had to be reached only after a period of time after discontinuing all OPV from the entire world – that was *en route* from Point B to Point C. Here is the inconvenient truth. OPV was not one of the safest of vaccines, but the only unsafe vaccine public health programs such as EPI was using -- and now the polio eradication was totally dependent on an unsafe vaccine.

It is no mystery then that a 12-year journey has taken 32 years and still has not reached anywhere near our destination, Point C. We cannot reach Point C without reaching Point B; at Point B we had to change tactics – OPV should no longer have been allowed anywhere in the world. Only IPV could be used. The journey from Point B to C will require at least three years, the minimum interval to feel confident that all chains of transmission of polioviruses, particularly vaccine viruses, are interrupted. In practical terms five years would be realistic. That means five years to 2000, namely 1995, should have been the chronological checkpoint, Point B, to have discontinued OPV in all low income countries – that is if the program was serious about global polio eradication by 2000. Now, in 2020, the increasing problem of cVDPV-2 is the continuing alarm bell to recommend the full immunising schedule of IPV, minimum two, optimum three doses, and get back on the path to reach Point B as early as possible.

The magnitude of poliovirus circulation in 2019 and 2020

In the case of wild polioviruses, among 200 children infected with WPV-1 only one child develops polio but the rest have silent infection. Among 1000-2000 children infected with WPV-2, only one develops polio.

In the case of circulating vaccine-derived polioviruses (cVDPV), their neurovirulence is intermediate between vaccine viruses and wild viruses -- nearer to vaccine viruses as they are derived from them. There is no data on the case-to-infection ratios. For cVDPV-1, one among 2000 to 20,000 infected would get polio – so we may assume. For cVDPV-2, one among 10,000 to 100,000 would get polio.

In 2019 and 2020, globally there were 366 and 857 cases of cVDPV-2 polio, respectively. They represent a huge number that were silently infected. Also in 2019 and 2020, there were 12 and 19 cases of cVDPV-1 polio, respectively, again representing orders of magnitude higher numbers of silent infections. Based on the detected cVDPV cases and the case:infection ratios, we can estimate the magnitude of the silent epidemics of cVDPV-1 and cVDPV-2.

The magnitude of cVDPV-1 epidemics was, thus, in the range of 38,000 – 380,000 in 2020. In 2019 it was between 24,000 and 240,000. The magnitude of cVDPV-2 epidemics in 2019 was between 3,660,000 and 36,600,000. The magnitude in 2020 was between 8,570,000 and 85,700,000.

For minimizing the consternation we get while eye-balling the magnitude of man-made polio, we take the most conservative case:infection ratios of 1:2000 for cVDPV-1 and 1:10,000 for cVDPV-2. With this assumption we calculate the minimum likely numbers of the total infections in the African continent and Asian continent and Table 9.1 presents the data. All cVDPV cases were in these two continents because most of the countries that use OPV very widely are in these two continents. The continent of South America does have many countries still using OPV, but the true annual statistics of polio vaccine-lineage viruses are not available to us. All countries in North America use IPV exclusively and have no VDPV polio.

Our conservative estimate shows that in 2019 more than 3.5 million and in 2020 more than 8.5 million children, respectively, were infected with vaccine-lineage poliovirus type 1 (cVDPV-1) or type 2 (cVDPV-2).

It is for this reason that we introduced the mental picture of 'house on fire' at the beginning of this chapter. The program is now looking for water to put the fire out and is beginning to dig a well, by way of hoping to get a novel type 2 vaccine -- moving from the laboratory to clinical trials and then to seek and hope for regulatory approvals from the many countries in need of dousing the fire. Finally, the hope is that the nOPV-2 will come to rescue the reputation of oral polio vaccine. The public ought to realize these issues, and either resign themselves to fate, or, become proactive and bring in realism into the global endeavor to eradicate all polioviruses.

Table 9.1 *Cases of polio caused by circulating vaccine-derived polioviruses, cVDPV1 and cVDPV2 and estimated total numbers of infection by cVDPV1 and cVDPV2 in 2019 and 2020. Case to infection ratio is 1:200 for WPV1 and 1:1000 for WPV2. Since VDPVs are less neurovirulent, we assume that case to infection ratios will be 1:2000 for cVDPV1 and 1:10,000 for cVDPV2.*

cVDPV-1 Globally		2019	2020
	Cases	12	19
	Infections	24,000	38,000
cVDPV-2 Africa	Cases	305	477
	Infections	3,050,000	4,770,000
cVDPV-2 Asia	Cases	35	336
	Infections	350,000	3,360,000

The future course cVDPV-1 and cVDPV-3 will take is unpredictable at present. The program is using widely bOPV with types 1 and 3 and these two vaccine viruses are unnecessarily getting seeded in too many countries. To interrupt cVDPV-2, many rounds of monovalent OPV type 2 (mOPV-2) were conducted in many countries and – got the house on more fire, by trying to put out fire with fire.

This is not the time to make more gambles by the program. Global polio eradication is precision public health, like putting man on the moon. If the scientists are not sure how to bring back the space vehicle with the explorers, they should not have ventured to take a shot at the moon.

The program must play safe assuming that cVDPV-1 and cVDPV-3 will pose problems in the future. All three viruses must be addressed together and for that novel OPVs against the three types is not the answer, but IPV is. A bird in hand is worth two in the bush; a vaccine in hand is worth more than two in the laboratory. We propose some practical tips for the way forward in Chapter 10.

Summation

Thirty-two years after the start of the global polio eradication program, twenty-five countries had polio outbreaks in 2020. However, natural polio cases are in only two countries among them. Man-made polio, in other words polio caused by vaccine-lineage viruses, are in all twenty-five countries. If there was no eradication program, we could be pleased that polio was reduced in the world – instead of 120 countries at the starting point, only 25 countries have polio in 2020.

However there are two major problems. One, the World Health Assembly launched the eradication program in 1988; eradication means that not even one child should suffer polio paralysis. That goal is out of reach, even out of sight, as of today. Hence the program is wandering and not on track. Second, the large majority of polio cases are not due to the viruses that were under eradication plan, but due to viruses newly introduced into communities by the program itself. These failures overshadow the successes of the program. Natural (wild) virus type 2 was eradicated in 1999, but the majority of polio cases now are due to vaccine virus type 2. No public health program has the right or even freedom to cause such harm in children. The ethical problem thus created is untenable any longer.

All polio today is in low income countries while all rich countries enjoy full freedom from polio. This inequity has been created by the eradication program; it goes against the spirit of public health. We compare the eradication program to a journey with a starting point and a well-defined goal that may be likened to a finishing line or destination. The travel had to reach a checkpoint in between to know that the journey is on track. The program has not yet reached that checkpoint. However, we have the knowledge and the tools to bring the journey back on track. Wisdom and determination are needed for continuing the journey to the finishing line.

The time to dig a well to find water is not when the house is on fire. This fire did not start accidentally. Who set the house on fire?

§§§

10. THE WAY FORWARD, CREATING A POLIO-FREE WORLD

"The winds and the waves are always on the side of the ablest
navigator" Edmund Gibbon

All is not lost. The eradication program can still be rescued and repaired towards assured success. To make the whole world polio-free, the program needs to accept some inconvenient truths, and, to approve appropriate remedies for the problems. The program at present appears to be drifting, not knowing how to go forward. The program now wants a new oral poliovirus vaccine type 2 to protect children against the circulating vaccine-derived poliovirus type 2 that was widely seeded by the program itself.

That is an unwise, expensive and time-consuming approach that has no guarantee of success, not even global acceptance of a new oral polio vaccine. Ethics, economic realism and epidemiological evidences demand that the program ought not procrastinate its completion and conclusion any longer.

The guidance inherent in the original World Health Assembly Resolution must be strictly adhered to. The program must realise that polio eradication, costing very heavy investments in money and human resources, had intended some spin off benefits – such as a strengthened Expanded Program on Immunisation and establishment of universal access to primary healthcare and promotion of essential diagnostic laboratory support. Polio eradication was supposed to be a vehicle for giving ride to these tangential and perhaps more valuable cargo – global public health leaders must regroup and decide whether or not these goals remain valid in the third decade of the twenty-first century.

Analysis of the paralysis

When the global polio eradication program was kick-started in 1988, there were two visible problems and one potential but invisible problem that EPI was facing regarding OPV and polio. The visible problems in all OPV-using countries were: one, high prevalence of wild polioviruses partly due to very low vaccine efficacy (failure of vaccine) of OPV and partly due to low OPV coverage (failure to vaccinate); and second, vaccine virus polio, called VAPP, in hundreds of children annually. Failure to vaccinate could be remedied, but failure of vaccine could not be remedied easily. Even VAPP could be prevented with at least one dose of IPV prior to OPV.

The invisible problem was known only to polio scientists, and most of them seem to have kept it as secret among themselves for far too long a time, to be helpful to lay leaders of the eradication partnership. The problem was: vaccine viruses spreading among children and becoming virulent enough to cause paralytic polio. If that became reality, by actually causing even polio outbreaks, then the mistake of keeping the information as secret would become embarrassingly exposed.

That is exactly what has happened in the last two decades, when outbreaks of polio due to circulating vaccine-derived polioviruses (cVDPV) have emerged to haunt the program. The man-made polio by far outnumbers natural wild-virus polio. That is untenable for an eradication program. Now scientists and lay leaders who brought the world to this situation are answerable to the thousands of paralyzed children, their families, their countries and all the donors who kept on donating without ensuring their donations were spent to end all polio, not to create polio.

Why did donors turn a Nelson's eye on the problem since 2000, without independently getting the problems in the program evaluated, in spite of long-standing and many times repeated advice to that effect? A list of fifteen publications that pointed out various issue relevant to this need for independent exploration of the problems and solutions, spanning from 1993 through 2016 is available.[1-15]

What is the reason for vaccine polio viruses turning wild-like? The reason consists of two undesirable properties of vaccine viruses, namely, transmissibility and genetic instability tending for back-mutation to virulence.[16] An acceptable live virus vaccine should be non-transmissible and genetically stable without genetic back-mutation that leads to de-attenuation. All live virus vaccines, right from smallpox vaccine, Pasteur's rabies vaccine and Theiler's yellow fever vaccine, to modern measles, mumps, rubella, varicella, rotavirus and hepatitis A vaccines, are virtually non-transmissible and essentially genetically stable without back-mutation to regain virulence. Live poliovirus vaccine is the exception – it is both transmissible and genetically reversible to virulence. It will not pass a vaccine trial for safety and efficacy in any tropical developing country.

The risk of vaccine polioviruses reacquiring the two parental properties that were markedly reduced during attenuation – hence unsafe for human use -- was known to all polio scientists. Essentially it was the phenomenon of de-attenuation, vaccine viruses turning wild-like under certain natural circumstances. Transmission enhanced the likelihood of back-mutation and back-mutation enhanced transmissibility. The result is vaccine viruses among children that cause contact-VAPP, community-acquired VAPP, sporadic polio due to VDPV (which is the same as community-acquired VAPP), polio due to iVDPV in immunodeficient children and adults, and ultimately outbreaks of polio due to circulating VDPV.

African countries altogether, or Africa as continent, was declared polio eradicated in the year 2019, full three years after the last case of wild virus polio in Nigeria. What is in very small print is that twenty one countries in Africa had polio outbreaks in 2020. The latter is not counted as polio by the program because they were polio cases created by the program – specifically due to cVDPV. Not calling it polio is to obfuscate the truth, which is of dubious propriety either in science or in ethics. Africa is not yet polio-free. Hundreds of African children had polio in 2019 and 2020.

In the previous chapter we described Points A, B and C. Has Africa reached Point C? No, polio is still widely prevalent. Has Africa reached Point B? No, OPV is still in widespread use in all countries in Africa. When was Africa due to decide it had reached Point B when OPV had to be discontinued? That is debatable, but we argue for end-2002, three years after wild poliovirus type 2 was globally eradicated by October 1999, following the three-year rule set by the program.[10] When was that certified? In 2014 – the question that needs asking is: why this delay of fifteen years when 3 years had been sufficient to know for sure if the virus had been eradicated? Had Point B been assigned in 2003 and only IPV was used in all countries since then, Point C could have been reached perhaps in another five years (2008-2009), or a couple of years more, by 2010 or 2011.

Now that vaccine-caused polio is rampant in Africa, ethics demands replacement of OPV with IPV as soon as possible. There is extreme urgency since the house is on fire – 19 countries had polio in 2019 and 25 countries in 2020. In other words, the way forward is to introduce IPV in EPI now, and ramp up its delivery country by country, and as high coverage is reached in any country, to ramp down and discontinue OPV. When all countries have only IPV and no more OPV in use, that will take the African continent to Point B. When the last of VDPV polio is past, Point C will have been reached.

The paralysis caused by de-attenuated vaccine virus could easily be mistaken for wild virus induced, unless the genetic sequence was analyzed. That is why we named it a potential but invisible problem in 1988 -- before genetic characterization was applied to every poliovirus from children's stools or from sewage.

Its earliest signal of this phenomenon was 'community-acquired VAPP', documented in countries with good disease surveillance and epidemiology expertise as early as 1964. The vaccine virus had to be circulating in the community for community acquisition -- by those who got infected – those who had neither been vaccinated nor had any contact with any vaccinated individual. Hence, the infection had to be due to vaccine viruses in circulation. As infection caused polio, the virus was obviously neurovirulent. Put two and two together and we get what we now call cVDPV.

VAPP in the vaccinated was no mystery: there is an inevitable but minuscule amount of neurovirulent polioviruses in every dose of OPV.[17,18] Back mutation begins when the Sabin strains are grown in cell culture to prepare OPV; hence back-mutated virus is inevitable in every dose. This fact was well known only among polio scientists.

What did VAPP in contacts of the vaccinated prove? It proved that vaccine viruses were transmissible. The fact of transmission of vaccine viruses to contacts was known to everyone, starting from Albert Sabin. However, how many generations of transmission, person to person, could occur with vaccine viruses? This question was not answered directly but was answered indirectly that it could occasionally continue in transmission until it circulated, proved by community-acquired VAPP. This was a crucial clue to the future potential but as yet invisible risk of vaccine viruses turning wild-like and turning the table on attempts to eradicate wild viruses with OPV. This once invisible problem is now all too obvious, and embarrassingly too frequent, virtually paralyzing the eradication program. In 2020 as of 20 December, 2 countries had wild virus polio (total 139 cases) while 25 countries had VDPV polio (total 876). Thus, for every natural case of polio in Afghanistan or Pakistan, there were about six vaccine-caused polio in 25 countries, most of them in Africa.

The eradication program erred by focusing only on OPV, instead on polio, but ignored the two problems of OPV – VAPP and vaccine viruses turning wild-like. In 2000, the latter was given the name 'vaccine-derived poliovirus' or VDPV. The program should have focused on polio, and preventing all polio, whether caused by wild virus or vaccine virus.

Ignoring VAPP, even though unethical as we have argued in chapter 8, could have been justified in the beginning but only for putting out the fire of polio outbreaks raging in many low-income countries in 1988. That deliberate and hard-hearted decision to place ethics on the back burner could only have been justified with the promise of its early withdrawal, as we reached Point B as described in Chapter 9-- on account of the fact VAPP would not be seeded any more when all OPV was withdrawn.

When should have all OPV been withdrawn, was then the critical question, and we have discussed it earlier and will repeat it later in this chapter. The program had planned withdrawal only after eradicating wild viruses globally, which was too risky, most unwise and simply unethical. Today the program is on the horns of a dilemma – to continue with OPV the way it is done now, or to protect every child using IPV – at least two doses – against all polio, vaccine-induced, or caused by cVDPV. No child gets polio after getting two well-timed doses of IPV. IPV is that exquisitely efficacious. On the other hand there was a child with lab proven polio in India after taking 50 doses of OPV.

The reason behind ignoring the signal of community-acquired VAPP (caused by VDPV circulating in the community), was, and remains, unexplained. It could not have been due to ignorance. It could have been only due to bias – favouring OPV and devaluing IPV. In that case, the program gambled on the risk, wishing that luck would be on their side – after all, eradication was for the good of generations of children.

As the probability of vaccine viruses regaining simultaneously the two properties lost in attenuation – transmission efficiency and neurovirulence -- was very low, the expectation might have been that wild viruses could be rapidly eradicated globally with OPV and all OPV could be withdrawn quickly, before that potential risk became real and visible to the public. That gamble would have been successful if eradication was achieved within a decade from the start and OPV withdrawn by 2000. The gamble failed, and VDPV problem exploded in 2006 because OPV was not withdrawn when it should have been withdrawn. There was one VDPV outbreak in Egypt prior to 1990 and one in Hispaniola Island in 2000, and none recognized from 2001 to 2005. That was the calm before the storm.

However, even if the risk might truly have been perceived as of very low probability, the consequence would be very bad. Wise judgment was needed to choose between completely safe intervention and intervention with a risk of low probability but high adverse impact. Gambling on it was a sign of bias and hubris. Wild polioviruses could not be eradicated rapidly and all OPV could not be withdrawn before or by 2000 – so the calculation went wrong.

The consequence of that failed gamble, namely, too many polio outbreaks in too many countries due to VDPVs, is today one of two major problems faced by the program. The *potential* problem became *real*; the *invisible* became *obvious*. Science explains; good science also *predicts*. What science predicted was apparently *believed* to be unlikely by the program experts. Depending on faith and luck was unscientific and unwise. Eradication was too serious a business to have been entrusted with polio fighters, mostly epidemiologists and public health professionals, all full of unrealistic optimism, hubris as we said earlier.

The second major problem currently faced by the program is antipathy to OPV in two countries – Afghanistan and Pakistan -- resulting in obstacles to reaching all children with repeated doses of OPV. Consequently, these two countries continue with circulating wild poliovirus type 1. Antipathy is only towards OPV, not any other vaccines. The reason for the antipathy must be explored. Unless the reason is understood, the way forward will remain foggy and unclear. Once the reason is understood, remedial steps will become clear.

Antipathy had originated in Nigeria in 2003 and spread to India, Afghanistan and Pakistan soon thereafter. In India and Nigeria, the problem could be mitigated and wild virus elimination was achieved. It may not be possible to overcome it in Afghanistan and Pakistan. In Pakistan, the animosity towards OPV had turned violent and inhuman -- with tragic outcomes: between December 2012 and July -2017, more than 100 health workers involved in polio immunization had been shot dead.[19] One government hospital in Peshawar district was burned down for administering OPV to children.[20] Even if the problem of obstacles to polio immunization with OPV is not solved, the program must be rescued – the way forward must be assured of success.

The situation in 2019 and 2020

All three problems mentioned above continue even in 2019 and 2020, but their importance has switched places. In the early years, wild viruses were the most important problem, but today VDPVs are the most important problem. Polio outbreaks due to VDPVs have affected 19 countries in 2019 and 25 countries in 2020, while wild poliovirus outbreaks continue to occur in only two countries. Wild polioviruses could be blocked with OPV, but OPV itself is the cause for the emergence of VDPVs, not merely for VAPP. Thus OPV is obviously incompatible with polio eradication.

If we depend on OPV for wild virus eradication, OPV from the vial must be given to all children repeatedly in OPV-using countries in order to keep VDPVs at bay. Vaccine viruses from the vaccine vial are far less transmissible and far less neurovirulent than VDPVs. However, the widespread feeding of OPV from the vials results in occasional VAPP in the vaccinated and their contacts as well as community-acquired VAPP, and the perpetuation of risks of VDPV emergence and VDPV circulation. Catch 22, as we said earlier.

Simple withdrawal of OPV after reaching zero wild virus polio in the community, in order to avoid all VAPP, is not safe as it enhances both the risk of the emergence of VDPVs and the risk of spread of emerged or imported VDPVs.

The story of Mogilev, well known to all polio scientists, is relevant here. In Mogilev, a region of the Byelorussian Republic of the former Soviet Union, an experiment was conducted to study the duration of protection created in the community by high coverage of OPV; the design was to stop all OPV and watch for subsequent events.[21]

The story was re-visited and described in detail with state of the art laboratory methods, after global polio eradication efforts had stalled, and published as a scientific paper in the reputed Journal of Virology, in 2003.[22]

We quote from that paper: *"We describe here a retrospective analysis of the cessation of OPV usage in a region of the Byelorussian Republic of the former Soviet Union in 1963 to 1966. During this period a widespread circulation and evolution of independent lineages of vaccine-derived polioviruses took place in the Region. Some of these lineages appeared to originate from OPV given to 40 children in the community during this period of essentially no vaccination. The data demonstrate very high risks associated with both the local cessation of OPV vaccination and the proposed use of OPV to control a possible resurgence of poliovirus in the post-vaccination period. The high transmissibility of OPV-derived viruses in non-immune population demonstrated here and the known existence of long-term OPV excretors should be also considered in assessing risks of the synchronised global cessation of OPV use."*

The resurgence of polio due to vaccine-derived virus was predominantly type 2. As we had said earlier, the withdrawal of type 2 from tOPV after wild type 2 was globally eradicated, was proposed for good reasons – to remove the vaccine that was no longer needed but was causing VAPP, and, to learn lessons for the future, when the withdrawal of types 3 and 1 will become necessary. In Mogilev, not only type 2 but also type 1 and type 3 had resurfaced. Instead of implementing the withdrawal of type 2 virus from tOPV in 2003, four years after eradication of wild virus type 2, it was postponed to 2016, seventeen years after eradication. In 2003, the background of community immunity would have been high since wild type 2 circulation had continued till a few years earlier and since tOPV coverage had reached a peak as evidenced by the eradication of wild virus type 2.

As foretold in Mogilev, type 2 vaccine-derived virus lineages began appearing and spreading in some countries from early 2006. In spite of the very clear warning not to re-introduce the removed vaccine virus type, the program resorted to fighting type 2 VDPVs with re-introduction of type 2 vaccine as a monovalent vaccine. The situation in 2019 and 2020, when the greater problem is VDPV type 2, than wild virus type 1, was created on account of the neglect of scientific data, prediction and cautionary advice.

One day the program will face the need to withdraw type 3 and also type 1 from OPV. Wild type 3 virus was last seen in the word in 2012. The program may decide to withdraw one type at a time or withdraw both types together. The Mogilev report has cautioned that even these vaccine virus types tend to remain in the community after withdrawal – and pose the risk of emergence of VDPVs types 1 and 3. Once withdrawn, the vaccine virus(es) should never be re-introduced.

There is only one safe way to withdraw OPV – and that is under cover of IPV immunization. This is not a new revelation – this was known to polio scientists all along, right from 1988, even earlier.

With this background information, designing a way forward to complete and conclude polio eradication is not very complicated. Some 150 countries are still using OPV and safely transitioning them from OPV to IPV is the only way forward for global polio eradication. That way, the two problems will be reduced to only one – that of wild type 1 poliovirus in Afghanistan and Pakistan. As the antipathy to OPV will be irrelevant once OPV is removed, even wild virus circulation can be, and must be, interrupted with IPV in these two countries. There is no alternate way for the program to proceed forward and succeed.

Hardcore polio virologists are working hard to create a new type 2 OPV – novel OPV (nOPV) with genetically modified virus strains that will be more stable than Sabin virus type 2.[23] Such an OPV will minimise the risk of the emergence of VDPVs. However, it will not overcome the antipathy against OPV in Afghanistan and Pakistan. There may be a future use of the nOPV2-CD. Meanwhile there cannot be any excuse for not including IPV in EPI – at least two doses or at most three doses. Already one dose is required in all countries that still use OPV. One more dose is what is needed, or at most two more doses.

In laboratory studies the newest version of such a virus, nOPV2-CD, performs quite well.[24] The scientists who developed and tested it in the laboratory have made a categorical assertion: "With the inherent inability to interrupt transmission, IPV alone is not the solution."[24] The problem for which the solution is said to be unsuitable is the spreading epidemics of cVDPV 2 in 25 countries in 2020 (until 23 December). Nine countries -- Afghanistan, Cameroun, Congo, Cote d'Ivoire, Guinea, Mali, Sierra Leon, Sudan, and South Sudan got newly affected with cVDPV-2 in 2020, with no such infection detected in the recent years past.

Against such a crisis situation, the program cannot wait any longer to develop, field test, obtain national regulatory approvals, manufacture and then for mass application. These steps will require an unknown period of time, a few years at a minimum. Even then registration in all countries may not happen. The program had taken 'gambles' in the past and failed every single time. Yet another gamble with the whole eradication program suspended on a thread of hope, not in the short term, but medium term at best, is most unwise.

Moreover, there is no supportive study or evidence for the assertion, that IPV alone is not the solution, which is merely an assumption, based on pre-existing beliefs and biases as we have shown in earlier chapters. IPV alone has been highly successful in many studies, in many countries. Why was the experimental switch to IPV from OPV made in Yogyakarta in Indonesia (we shall discuss this further in the next section) ? Why doesn't the program apply the results of that study in the program?

Circulating VDPV type 1 is also a potential future problem. If we chase only cVDPV-2 now and cVDPV-1 becomes a problem, then what is its solution? IPV will cover all three virus types.

Where evidence and logic are absent, dogma cannot be their surrogate. IPV alone is the solution. Introduction of IPV in EPI is an urgent necessity -- now, as it is already many years too late. Ethics demands it; epidemiology supports it; economics is most probably positive. Even if some people do not expect IPV to interrupt transmission, no one can honestly argue that polio paralysis should not be prevented in every single child, for which giving two to three doses of IPV is the solution already available. When IPV coverage is built up to 85% to 90%, VDPV will die out. For the sake of argument, the nOPV can still be used in campaign mode in case the VDPV does not die out. So, let research continue but research should not hold up eradication drive using the available and exquisitely efficacious vaccine, IPV.

Is the program more interested in somehow defending the reputation of OPV than eradicating polio? However, the new OPV will not be Sabin OPV; Sabin OPV's reputation cannot be rescued by the new genetically modified OPV, even it becomes a reality. Oliver Goldsmith wrote in his poem, The Village Schoolmaster: *"e'en though vanquished, he could argue still."*

Wild viruses must be eliminated now using a fully immunizing schedule of IPV in EPI in Afghanistan and Pakistan. OPV to IPV transition is urgently needed in these two countries on a priority basis. The program must learn to control and eliminate wild virus polio, which requires the strengthening of EPI. When diphtheria, pertussis and measles are targeted for control, for which EPI vaccines are essential, IPV can be 'smuggled in' as combination vaccine, without upsetting anyone. The EPI schedule is with 3 doses and three doses of the IPV-containing vaccine will probably be welcomed by those who oppose OPV.

The wise drafters of the 1988 Resolution wanted eradication that way, through EPI. Transition to IPV is also needed, as soon as possible, in all other OPV-using countries as well.

The remaining question for the eradication program is whether such transition should be planned for all 150 OPV-using countries simultaneously, or if the transition can be planned in a staggered manner – staggered by WHO Regions or staggered by individual countries.

Could OPV-to-IPV transition be staggered by Regions?

The Region of the Americas was certified polio-free in August 1994, Western Pacific in October 2000, Europe in June 2002 and SE Asia in March 2014.[25] The program recognises only wild virus polio as polio – hence polio eradicated was only partly true. However, even after certification, the program has not transitioned any of these Regions from OPV to IPV. The most likely message is that the program is waiting to achieve the elimination of wild viruses globally before such a transition is considered in all OPV-using countries in all Regions.

The program does not manufacture IPV or OPV. The world is dependent on commercial (or state-owned) manufacturers. Up-scaling production to meet any volume of demand is easier for OPV, monovalent or bivalent, than for IPV. As the eradication program had excluded IPV from its policy and plan from the beginning, the number of IPV manufacturers had dwindled to only a few players. Under these circumstances, simultaneous transition in all Regions will not be feasible as of today or in the immediate future. The staggered transition will be feasible – market volume needs to expand only gradually. Is there any risk involved in a staggered transition?

The possible risk is for the trans-country spread of vaccine viruses or VDPVs from countries in Regions not yet transitioned from OPV to IPV to countries that have already transitioned. Such risks are real, but their probabilities depend on many factors – risk will be very small if high IPV coverage is achieved prior to withdrawing OPV. There have been many instances in which VDPVs had been imported into IPV-using countries, but in no instance did the VDPVs cause polio outbreak or circulate for long. If importation is detected, it should be put down only with more IPV, never with OPV. Let us examine the six WHO Regions.

The vast majority of countries in the Region of Europe are already using IPV exclusively. Only a small number of countries need to introduce IPV in their immunization schedule in order to wean the Region from OPV. But their population size is not small. As they all are high-income countries, with high immunization coverage, the transition should be programmatically and technically easy. There need be no delay for articulating the policy for the transition. What is needed is the policy of the program.

In the Region of Americas, the transition will be easier, as the population size of countries now on OPV is smaller than those using only IPV and as all countries have very robust immunization programs achieving very high coverage. In fact, immunization coverage is so high that measles and rubella transmission was interrupted in the entire Region. There need be no delay for the policy shift towards implementing the transition.

In the Western Pacific Region, China, the country with the largest population in the world, tilts the balance between OPV and IPV. However, very wisely Chinese vaccine manufacturers are ready to roll out IPV (made by inactivating Sabin strains of attenuated polioviruses instead of wild polioviruses) to fully meet national needs. Only a clear policy signal from the program remains for the national policy to move forward with the transition. Seven of the 27 countries in the Region are already on exclusive IPV regime. Here also transition will be easy; it must begin with the policy shift, for which there should be no delay.

These three are the Regions that had set goals of polio elimination ahead of the 1988 WHA Resolution for global eradication. These same three Regions could prove to the world the feasibility and realism in completing and concluding polio elimination – wild, vaccine, and vaccine-derived. The world deserves to be encouraged by such good news.

In South-East Asia Region, none among the 11 countries is on IPV regimen. Interestingly, one province in Indonesia, that of Yogyakarta (population 3.5 million), has been using IPV exclusively since September 2007, as an experiment – while neighbouring districts and the rest of the country continue using OPV.[26] Yogyakarta has been free of all polio for the entire period till now. So, a staggered transition is quite safe without fear of its effectiveness and safety. Neither vaccine viruses nor vaccine-derived viruses have invaded Yogyakarta all these years, attesting to the robustness of immunity provided by IPV.

Why was that *experiment* designed and conducted? Obviously, it was to see if it would be safe and successful to transition from OPV to IPV in one large geographic population – we laud and applaud the vision of those who designed and implemented the *experiment*. But we bemoan the neglect of its logical follow-up action. Indonesia, we understand, is likely to transition to IPV as soon as the polio vaccine manufacturing facility in Bandung is able to produce enough IPV for the whole country.

India, the country with the second largest population in the world had once successfully manufactured IPV in Pune in Maharashtra State, but national policy disallowed continued production. [27] A large IPV manufacturing facility was initiated in the Delhi Capital region, in 1987, one year prior to the Eradication Resolution, as Indian biomedical scientists had understood its need in India. The OPV-only policy was felt to be unwise on account of very low efficacy of OPV plus its safety problem. Just before production was to start, the initiative was abruptly aborted – under rather mysterious circumstances. We understand that it was due to the influence of the program policy of exclusive use of OPV. Had that facility been allowed to manufacture IPV, the whole world, not only India, would have benefited immensely. Currently, one multinational manufacturer with its filling and distributing plant in India produces a large volume of IPV and exports it all to other countries, as the national policy does not demand IPV for a transition from OPV.

In the Region of Africa, wild poliovirus transmission was certified interrupted in 2016, just over three years ago. While the countries in the Regions of Americas, Europe, Western Pacific and South East Asia could largely absorb the costs involved for the transition, with continuing assistance from the program for monitoring and surveillance, many if not most of the 45 countries in Africa Region will need external financial support for the OPV to IPV transition.

This is where the program must invest its resources without reservation. The problem of polio outbreaks due to cVDPV is most severe in Angola, Central African Republic, Democratic Republic of Congo, Ghana, Cote d'Ivoire, Burkina Faso, Sudan, Nigeria, Mali, Togo, Ethiopia and Somalia – all in this Region. It is here the OPV-IPV transition is most urgently needed but perhaps the most difficult to implement. The earlier the process starts, the better for the Region and the whole world.

The urgency to transition from OPV to IPV is obviously in the Africa Region which is on cVDPV fire. The program and all donor agencies must understand this reality and work out the necessary war-room plans to achieve it.

Last, the Eastern Mediterranean Region, which has 20 countries, some of which are among the richest in the world and some among the poorest. Two countries – Afghanistan and Pakistan – have not yet interrupted wild poliovirus type 1. The animosity to OPV in them is not abating. The prospects of eliminating wild poliovirus type 1 are getting dimmer every year. The obstinacy of the OPV-only policy of the program is self-defeating and unnecessary – we say, even foolhardy. In these two countries, the transition is very urgent. Here OPV, Sabin OPV or a new *avatar* novel OPV, is like *'red rag in front of the bull'* – IPV, given as combination vaccine – quadrivalent with DPT and IPV or hexavalent with DPT, IPV, Hepatitis B antigen and *Haemophilus influenzae* b antigen, should replace IPV as soon as possible. Remember, no child has developed polio after 'full immunization' with IPV. Two well-timed doses or three doses given by conventional EPI schedule constitute full immunization.

If wild poliovirus transmission must be interrupted using OPV, near-100% coverage with many repeated doses, at least 7-10 doses per child, in some countries more than 20 doses, will be necessary. That is why it had taken an inordinate number of years in India and Nigeria to eliminate wild viruses; in Afghanistan and Pakistan, it has not been possible to eliminate wild virus polio type 1 while programmatic deficiencies are compounded with obstacles due to antipathy against OPV. If IPV is used, 2-3 doses per child, and at best some 80-85% coverage, at worst 90-95% achieved, if coverage is evenly distributed, may suffice to interrupt transmission. IPV offers much higher herd effect than OPV. Why has the program not investigated, or learned from others, this important lesson? It is in this background that the program should re-visit the war room plans for elimination poliovirus infection, wild and vaccine-derived from community source, and vaccine viruses from vaccine vials.

In short, for true polio eradication, the need for OPV to IPV transition is inevitable and 'non-negotiable' as there is no alternative to it; here we argue that it could be planned and implemented in a staggered manner, staggered by WHO Regions. Staggered transition is without undue risk and programmatically feasible. Transition, staggered or otherwise, is essential for the world to move forward from the rut it finds itself with polio outbreaks of vaccine-derived viruses in many countries. In case of any trans-country importation of polio, that must be countered with high coverage of IPV.

From pragmatic viewpoint and in the face of today's severe market constraints of IPV supply, such staggered transition is one obvious way forward. Another possibility is even simpler -- more decentralised – staggered by individual countries.

Could OPV-to-IPV transition be staggered by countries?

Today some 50 countries use IPV and have achieved true polio elimination – no infection with wild or vaccine viruses – and reached Point C several years ago. They belong to all six WHO Regions.

They live side by side with countries using OPV. They are visited by many individuals and families from countries with the continuing problem of polio, wild virus polio or VDPV polio. They have no VAPP, and they have a very low risk of importation of VDPVs or even vaccine viruses. Even if VDPV enters an IPV country, the probability of polio will be zero and that of spread will be quite low.

Therefore, it stands to reason that the OPV-IPV transition can be staggered by countries in different WHO Regions. This reasoning ought to be a great relief for the eradication program, for which a globally synchronous transition would be a nightmare. A transition staggered by Regions may face supply problems of IPV, which we hear is slowly abating. Enough supply for the whole world will take another two or three years.

There is no need to wait for that to happen before the policy shift is established, and the process of OPV-IPV transition is begun. This can begin only if a country-by-country transition is an assured, safe way forward. We have courage of conviction in its rationale to say it will be safe. A policy shift can happen immediately if the program leaders want polio eradication achieved in the shortest possible time.

What happened, or what did not happen, in neighbouring countries, when South Korea, Brunei and Malaysia switched to IPV, is a lesson for the program to plan and move forward to complete and conclude eradication expeditiously and without risk, by encouraging more countries to transition to IPV immunization schedule.

As mentioned above, an 'island' of exclusive IPV use was created in 2007, in Yogyakarta Province in Indonesia that uses only OPV in all other Provinces. Yogyakarta has been free of all polio for the entire period till date. Neither vaccine viruses nor vaccine-derived viruses have invaded Yogyakarta all these years, attesting to the robustness of immunity provided by IPV. So, staggered country by country transition is quite effective and quite safe.

Country-by-country transition is thus effective, safe and feasible. What stands in its way? Simply, the inflexible program policy. If the program could announce a policy that allows countries to switch to IPV, that will have an immediate effect as well as a domino effect, and we can hope for early completion of polio eradication.

A policy shift will enable countries to feel comfortable to transition from OPV to IPV. For example, India could demand that the multinational manufacturer that operates in

India first fulfil India's needs before exporting IPV to other countries.

Middle East countries use IPV in their children for their best interests and also OPV, ostensibly to comply with eradication program's policy. If the policy provides freedom for countries to transition to IPV, such countries may feel comfortable to transition to an all IPV immunization schedule against polio and to discontinue OPV use currently used for pleasing the program.

Vaccine manufacturers will hopefully meet comfortably with such country-by-country increase in demand for IPV, which would be more gradual than Regional demand for many countries at one time.

When all countries transition to IPV and OPV use is discontinued, the world would have reached 'Point B' of the diagram in Chapter 9 and got closer to the eradication goal and finish line. Globally, except in Afghanistan and Pakistan, all other countries will have stopped introducing the second cause of polio, namely Sabin strains of polioviruses.

That is an essential milestone *en route* to reaching a polio-free world, that we called 'Point B' in Chapter 9. After reaching 'Point B', all remaining polio, whether wild virus-caused (in Afghanistan and Pakistan) or VDPV-caused (in many countries), ought to be eliminated only with IPV. When no OPV is fed in the community, no new lineage of VDPV can emerge from vaccinated children. All lineages of VDPV that have already emerged and are circulating visibly or silently must be interrupted with IPV. Such silently circulating VDPVs may be detected through sewage surveillance where that is done, or through clinical and virological AFP surveillance alone, where sewage surveillance is not practiced.

We presume that in 2 or 3 years of exclusive use of IPV, a country, a Region, or, the entire the world, should reach 'Point C' described in Chapter 9 – without any poliovirus transmission, wild and vaccine. In the interim there may be vaccine-lineage virus in the community but no polio in any child with at least two doses of IPV. Such viruses tend to die out under sustained immunisation pressure of IPV.

If a policy shift for OPV-to-IPV transition is made in 2020, and all countries transition by last quarter of 2021, global eradication can succeed by last quarter of 2023 and be so certified in 2026. If one year for margin of error is allowed, eradication may be achieved in 2024 and certified in 2027. The beauty of IPV is that it is so efficacious that it is like a hot knife on frozen butter.

The history and geography of antipathy to OPV

The antipathy to OPV in Pakistan and Afghanistan is continuing, and continuing to seriously hurt the efforts to eliminate wild poliovirus type 1 from these two countries. There were 147 and 29 cases of type 1 polio in these two countries in 2019 respectively and 82 and 56 in 2020 (data as of 20th Dec 2020. As long as this antipathy continues, the prospects of success are very low, unless the tactics are shifted from total reliance on OPV to total reliance on IPV. We trace back the origins of the antipathy to OPV. It all started in northern Nigeria in 2003. Northern Nigeria is predominantly Muslim.

Since the Second World War, ill feelings of Muslims in the Middle East and West Asia towards the Western powers had festered as was well known to all. As the WHA Resolution to eradicate polio was passed unanimously in 1988, it was clear that Public Health had priority over political tensions all over the world, including that between Muslim countries and the rest, particularly the West. Had eradication been accomplished by the year 2000, all would have been well – politics would not have interfered with the program.

Nigeria had wild poliovirus types 1 and 3 continuing into the 21st century and the eradication program was desperately trying to catch up, unmindful of the drastically changing global scenario of the tensions mentioned above.

The original idea was to eradicate polio irrespective of the ground conditions of inequity in almost every welfare service in low-income countries. The vision of the leaders who drafted the 1988 WHA Resolution had most probably taken into account the mismatch between the healthcare needs of people in underserved communities and the potential of EPI to bridge that gap to a certain degree.

Polio eradication was to be achieved through EPI, suitably strengthened and streamlined. Wise leaders would have perceived the mismatch between what people wanted and what the program could deliver. Once polio was eradicated through EPI, the value of EPI would become appreciated by all low-income countries.

As the program divorced eradication from EPI, it was extremely important that success was achieved by 2000, before the several potential fault lines could become too serious and disruptive. The world changed in 2001, specifically on 11 Sept – with the infamous terrorism events of 9/11 in the USA, of unprecedented magnitude. Suspicion and trust deficit exploded. That was time for the program to be alert and sensitive.

In 2002 the USA invaded Iraq. That made many Muslims in many countries suspect that they were being targeted by the West. In northern Nigeria the question arose as to why polio was given exclusive importance -- why OPV was given free of cost and repeatedly many times to all under-five children while other EPI vaccines were neglected -- why health workers visited homes to give OPV but not for any other legitimate needs of families -- why girl children were given importance in the program. For polio eradication all of these were essential, but there was a trust deficit that was not addressed by the program implementers.

There were other reasons for Nigerians to be suspicious of the intentions of the program, led by many Western well-meaning personnel. In 1996 a USA-based pharmaceutical company had conducted a clinical trial in northern Nigeria using an experimental drug, trovafloxacin. The clinical trial had too many flaws, ethical and procedural, that made Nigerians believe that they were being unfairly used as guinea pigs. The experimental drug was being compared to the standard drug – but the dose of the standard drug had been pegged down presumably to render it less effective than with proper dosage. Court cases followed and eventually the company settled the matter out of court, the settlement amount was US$ 75 million.[28]

In 2001, between February and May, there was an outbreak of 100,000 children with measles. In this setting, *"polio vaccinators were seen as absurd and inappropriate as they entered houses to administer polio vaccines as parents mourned the deaths of their children from measles."*[29]

During 2001-2002, nearly half of all polio cases in the world and over three-quarters of all cases in Africa were in Nigeria. In mid-October 2003 the program launched an ambitious campaign to cover 15 million children in West and central Africa. Nigeria was the most important country for the campaign. The three worst-affected states in northern Nigeria boycotted the campaign.[30]

We quote from the paper by Jegede AS: "*Sule Ya'u Sule speaking for the governor of Kano, is quoted saying: since 11 Sept, the Muslim world is beginning to be suspicious of any move from the Western world... Our people have become really concerned about polio vaccine. Datti Ahmed, a Kano-based physician who heads a prominent Muslim group – the Supreme Council of Sharia in Nigeria is quoted as saying that polio vaccines were corrupted and tainted by evildoers from America and their Western Allies... We believe that modern-day Hitlers have deliberately adulterated the oral polio vaccines with anti-fertility drugs and viruses which are known to cause AIDS."*

"Another important factor that played a role in the polio vaccine boycott was the general distrust of aggressive mass immunization programs in a country where access to basic healthcare is not easily available...

From a Nigerian perspective, to be offered free medicine is about as unusual as a stranger's going door to door in America and handing over $ 100 bills. It does not make sense in a country where people struggle to obtain the most basic medicines and treatment at local clinics."[30]

What was the proximal provocation for the boycott? In 2003, among rumours and mistrust, the Government decided to get OPV tested for any deleterious substances. A Nigerian pharmacologist, Dr Alhassan Bichi, subjected OPV to spectroscopy and detected a low-level contaminant structurally similar to estradiol, a female hormone. He opined: *"when polio vaccine is seen to contain something that has not been declared, then I find it unethical to recommend that the vaccine be used"* (The vaccine used in Nigeria was then submitted to an Indian laboratory under WHO supervision). Hilary Butler, a freelance journalist, wrote that the Indian laboratory found the contaminants; the vaccine was grossly substandard and failed all tests of safety and purity.[31,32]. Eventually the crisis blew over; Nigerians accepted OPV manufactured in Indonesia, another Muslim country. The antipathy to OPV by Muslims spread to northern India, where it was handled superbly by the program personnel, supported by the Government and non-governmental agencies such as the Rotary. In Pakistan and Afghanistan problem was not solved and continues to this day.

The problem everybody saw was the program's OPV-centric behaviours, unmindful of its repercussions on polio eradication.

Will chronic vaccine-virus infections negate eradication?

Imagine the world that would have eradicated all transmission of polioviruses, wild and vaccine – quite possible earliest by 2023 if the program accepts the recommended policy shifts and program re-design in 2021, and so certified by the Global Polio Eradication Commission three years later, by 2026. In this scenario, all countries would have transitioned to an all IPV regimen by the end of 2022 or 2023. There would be, hopefully, zero 'incidence' (biomedical jargon for newly transmitted infection), of any poliovirus infection anywhere in the world.

A true case of polio, due to poliovirus, not wild, but vaccine-derived (more specifically immunodeficiency-associated VDPV, iVDPV), due to chronic infection and not fresh transmission – could still occur in someone somewhere in the world even after the certification of global polio eradication!

Chronic infections will continue to be prevalent on account of children with immune-deficiency of the 'B cells' of the immune system, who might have been fed OPV before its withdrawal in the year 2021. Such chronically infected individuals have a high probability of developing polio paralysis after months or years of chronicity of infection.

Such a case of polio will not negate the world status of polio eradication, since that case will not be due to 'incidence' of infection but due to 'prevalence' (jargon for infection already present in the community or in an individual) of Sabin virus infection. Eradication is zero 'incidence' of poliovirus infection – a pre-existing infection that qualifies for 'prevalence' is not under our eradication definition.

Obviously, the incidence of infection in the community, due to transmission from chronic virus shedding persons, must be prevented by maintaining high IPV coverage in the community. Once the whole world in under IPV coverage, such stray instances will be rare, but the program should be alert to detect it. After eradication, the program infrastructure may cease to exist – therefore all countries should be aware of this potential risk.

Immunization with IPV will have to continue at least until all such risks are behind us – which may take a number of years.

Risks of re-introduction of eradicated polioviruses may have other sources – leak from IPV manufacturing facilities, from stored virus stocks or virus containing human clinical samples kept in freezers or even malicious and intentional introduction, will continue. Therefore, we cannot know or predict how long the world should continue immunising against polio.

Summation

Polio eradication program must succeed, and succeed as early as possible. The goal of the program should be to achieve a polio-free world, qualified as 'zero incidence of poliovirus infection'. Incidence refers to new infection – no child or adult should get newly infected with poliovirus, wild, vaccine or vaccine-derived. There is no controversy regarding the need for zero incidence of wild poliovirus infection in the polio eradicated world. But the need to eradicate vaccine, vaccine-like and vaccine-derived viruses must be accepted by the program as the first step towards getting back on track towards success.

There are immune-deficient persons chronically infected with vaccine viruses and are shedding them in their faeces. They will continue to remain infected for months or years. In epidemiology parlance infection already present is called 'prevalence', not incidence as the infection is not new. As the goal is zero incidence, the prevalence of infection does not negate eradication status, but incidence due to transmission must be prevented. In other words, prevalent infection must not result in infection in anyone else in the family or community. For that purpose necessary sanitary precautions must in place to minimise the chance of transmission. All persons in the family and in the neighbourhood should be well protected by vaccination with IPV. In the unlikely event of transmission in the polio-eradicated world, it ought to be detected and further transmission averted, or, if in transmission it ought to be interrupted.

There may arise a paradoxical situation: a chronically infected person may develop polio paralysis. That may occur after the world has achieved zero incidence of poliovirus infection. It may occur after the world is certified polio eradicated. Such events will have to be expected and documented but they do not negate eradication status.

As OPV is incompatible with polio eradication, the checkpoint towards right track is the discontinuation of OPV vaccination under cover of IPV immunisation program. Because IPV was disallowed in low income countries for decades, the global supply of IPV is currently inadequate to cover the requirement of whole world. Therefore, IPV introduction and OPV withdrawal can only be planned in a staggered manner. The transition is named Point B. When all countries and Regions reach Point B without any OPV in use, the world would have reached the checkpoint. From then onwards only IPV should be in use, universally. That will be an equitable world, the rich and poor getting the safe IPV.

Beyond Point B in any country, the detection of any poliovirus in transmission must attract intensive IPV immunisation and no panic re-introduction of OPV under any circumstance. Under high IPV coverage, 85% to 90% by age 5 years, poliovirus transmission, WPV or vaccine-lineage, will die out. All polio outbreaks last about 6 months to one year; therefore the die out also is to be expected within such a time frame.

We can achieve global polio eradication, no doubt about it. We owe it to the world's new generations of children.

WHO can then help establish Public Health and Primary Healthcare, using funds saved from polio eradication, in all countries now practicing the Expanded Program on Immunisation. Every child deserves to be protected against all vaccine-preventable diseases.

§§§

EPILOGUE

We request the reader to refresh memory of the Preface and Parable, by reading them once again.

Imagine if we were two aliens visiting earth. Imagine we heard the story of the polio eradication program – its lofty ideals, the global partnerships, the liberal funding, and two vaccines against polio – but that the program has failed to achieve success in 2000, as the then leaders had wanted.

Twenty years later we the aliens ask the program leaders, why did you try to eradicate polio using only one of the two vaccines, and what is the answer?

You don't understand our rules. Here is an infection in the intestines and lots of virus shed in stools. We want the shedding of virus in stool stopped so that polio can be eradicated. The other vaccine does not induce sufficient intestinal immunity to stop the stool-shedding of the virus. That is our belief. One vaccine induces strong, even if very transient, intestinal immunity and that is the vaccine that will eradicate polio. That is our rule.

Aliens ask, if the vaccination by your rule failed to achieve polio eradication, could your rule be faulty?

No, never, we make rules based on what we believe so that the rules will guide us. The belief is sacred, so are the rules. They have been passed on to us by our Pundits and Gurus in the past.

The aliens had brains that worked more like those of rats. Rats learn by information integration and solve problems by it. Humans make rules and try to solve problems by their rules. This has been experimentally proved.[1] The aliens mused between them – these humans think they are the smartest animals on earth. They are more interested to stop poliovirus shedding in the stools of children rather than to prevent polio in children. They want to eradicate polio without using the vaccine that will predictably prevent polio in them but using the vaccine that reduces virus shedding in some children but does not protect the others from polio. And they don't mind if their sacred vaccine caused polio in some children. How strange. They made the rule by themselves and are obsessed with following their rule and in the process they have lost the goal of polio eradication. The aliens remembered what the psychiatrist AKM Nagaraj had once said: Human mind's greatest weakness is to make concepts that fit into its belief and then believe that this is the absolute truth.[2]

They don't see the glass wall between their belief and rule on one side and their mission on the other. All they want is to prove first that the rule they made based on belief was correct and later only they will move on to the real goal of polio eradication. That is inconsistent with our way of thinking by information integration. There are so many vaccines that are given by injection and they all reduce the spread of the microbes among people, whether the infection is intestinal or respiratory. Now we know: the rule is actually their glass wall. Others who use those other vaccines never made any such rule. They just observed without pre-conceived rule based on any belief. When they found exquisite herd effect of many injected vaccines like those against *Haemophilus influenzae b* or *pneumococci,* whooping cough or diphtheria, they just accepted that as fact and moved on. These polio people should not have made any rule, just observe facts. Faith in the rule is the reason why these program leaders cannot get the rule out of their mind and get on with polio eradication.

The aliens asked – where is smallpox virus shed?

In the respiratory secretions and that was why smallpox was contagious, spreading even by mere social contact with a case of smallpox.

Oh then you eradicated smallpox using a vaccine that was given via the nose, right?

No, you don't understand, the smallpox vaccine was inoculated on the skin.

Aliens asked: then what about your rule?

Sorry, smallpox was eradicated before we made our rule.

Aliens observed: we understand now, if you had only one vaccine that was inoculated through the skin, you could have eradicated polio long ago, and not make a rule that confused you.

The humans said: *no, we say a rule is a rule is a rule...*

The aliens said: get rid of your rule and you will succeed, we guarantee. Good luck, said they before moving on to enjoy the wonderful sights on the earth and to listen to the beautiful music the humans create. They tuned in and listened to: *Que Sera Sera, whatever will be will be.*

§§§

NOTES

Chapter 1 Declaring War on Polio: Revisiting the Resolution

1. Henderson DA. A history of eradication—successes, failures, and controversies. Lancet March 10, 2012; 379 (9819): 884-885.

2. Walsh J, Warren K. Selective Primary Health Care: an interim strategy for disdease control in developing countries New Eng J Med 1979; 18: 967-974

3. Newell KW. Selective Primary Health Care: The Counter Revolution Social Science and Medicine 1988; 26: 903–906

4. John TJ, Plotkin SA, Orenstein WA. Building on the success of the Expanded Programme on Immunisation: Enhancing the focus on disease prevention and control. Vaccine 2011; 29: 8835-8837.

5. UNESCO. The Talloires Declaration.10-12 March 1988. Available from https://www.unicef.org/about/history/files/Talloires_declaration_1988.pdf.

6. World Health Assembly. Forty-first World Health Assembly, Geneva, 2-13 MAY 1988. WHA41.28 Global eradication of poliomyelitis by the year 2000. Available from https://www.who.int/ihr/polioresolution4128en.pdf.

7. John TJ, Samuel R, Balraj V, John R. Disease surveillance at district level: a model for developing countries. Lancet 1998 Jul 4;352(9121):58-61.

8. John TJ, Rajappan K, Arjunan KK. Communicable diseases monitored by disease surveillance in Kottayam district, Kerala state, India. Indian J Med Res. 2004 Aug;120(2):86-93.

9. Pandey AA and Chandel S. Human resource assessment of a district hospital applying WISN method: Role of laboratory

technicians. International Journal of Medicine and Public Health. 2013;3(4):260-270.

10. Dowdle WR, Hopkins DR, editors. The Eradication of Infectious Diseases. New York: John Wiley & Sons; 1998. (Report of the Dahlem Workshop on the Eradication of Infection Diseases, Berlin, March 16–22, 1997).

11. Cratylus (dialogue) Accessed from https://en.wikipedia.org/wiki/Cratylus_(dialogue)#cite_note-12

12. Patel M, Shane AL, Parashar UD, Jiang B, Gentsch JR, Glass RI. Oral rotavirus vaccines: how well will they work where they are needed most?. *J Infect Dis.* 2009;200 Suppl 1(0 1):S39–S48. doi:10.1086/605035.

13. John TJ. Problems with oral poliovaccine in India. Indian Pediatr 1972; 9: 252-256.

14. Choudhari AR and Kumar D. Emergence of Modern Science in Colonial India. INSA New Delhi 2018.

15. Abraham T. Polio: the odyssey of eradication. London, Hurst and Co (Publishers) Ltd; 2018.

16. John TJ. Immunisation against poliovirus in developing countries. Rev Med Virol 1993; 3:149-160.

17. John TJ. Role of injectable and oral polio vaccines in polio eradication. Expert Rev Vaccines. 2009 Jan;8(1):5-8. doi: 10.1586/14760584.8.1.5.

Chapter 3 An instrument to compare vaccines, OPV and IPV

1. Melnick JL. Live attenuated poliovirus vaccines. Plotkin SA, Mortimer EA In Vaccines. 2nd ed. Philadelphia: Saunders; 1994, Chapter no.7, 129p.

2. Miller DL, Galbraith NS. Surveillance of the safety of oral poliomyelitis vaccine in England and Wales 1962-4. *Br Med J.* 1965; 2 (5460): 504-9.

3. WHO Consultative Group. The relation between acute persisting spinal paralysis and poliomyelitis vaccine--results

of a ten-year enquiry. Bull World Health Organ. 1982;60 (2):231-42.

4. John TJ. Problems with OPV in India. Indian Pediatrics 1972;9; 252- 256.

5. Ratnaswamy L, John TJ, Jadhav M. Paralytic poliomyelitis: clinical and virological studies. Indian Pediatr 1973; 10:443-447.

6. John TJ, Jayabal P. Oral polio vaccination of children in the tropics. Amer J Epidemiol 1972; 96: 263-269.

7. John TJ. Oral polio vaccination of children in the tropics. Antibody response in relation to vaccine virus infection. Am J Epidemiol 1975; 102:414-421.

8. John TJ, Christopher S. Oral polio vaccination of children in the tropics. Intercurrent enterovirus infection, vaccine virus take and antibody response. Am J Epidemiol 1975; 102: 422-428

9. John TJ.Towards a National policy on Poliomyelitis. Indian pediatrics 1981;18(8):503-506.

10. John TJ. Lessons from the polio eradication campaign. Seminar March 2012; 631: 16-20).

11. Prabakar N, Srilatha V, Mukerji D, John A, Rajarathnam A, John TJ.The epidemiology and prevention of poliomyelitis in a rural community in south India. Indian Pediatrics 1981 Aug;18(8):527-37.

12. Basu RN. Magnitude of problem of Poliomyelitis Indian pediatrics 1981;18(8):507-512.

13. John TK and John TJ. Is poliomyelitis a serious problem in developing countries? The Vellore experience; J. Trop. Pediatrics 1982(28): 11-16.

14. Joseph B, Ravikumar R, John M, Natarajan M, Steinhoff M C and John TJ. Comparison of techniques for the estimation of the prevalence of poliomyelitis in developing countries; Bull WHO 1983; 610: 833-837.

15. John TJ, Plotkin SA, Orenstein WA.Building on the success of the Expanded Programme on Immunization: enhancing

the focus on disease prevention and control.Vaccine. 2011 Nov 8;29(48):8835-7. doi: 10.1016/j.vaccine.2011.08.100. Epub 2011 Oct 3.

16. John TJ.Understanding the Scientific Basis of Preventing Polio by Immunization. Pioneering Contributions from India.Proc.Indian natn Sci Acad. 2003 ;B69 (4) :393-422.

17. Patriarca PA, Wright PF, John TJ. Factors affecting the immunogenicity of oral poliovirus vaccine in developing countries. Rev Infect Dis 1991; 13: 926-939.

18. The relation between acute persisting spinal paralysis and poliomyelitis vaccine (oral): results of a WHO enquiry. Bull World Health Organ. 1976;53(4):319-31.

19. Nkowane BM, Wassilak SGM, Orenstein WA et al. Vaccine-associated paralytic poliomyelitis. Unites States, 1973 through 1984. JAMA 1987; 257: 1335-1340.

20. Yang CF, Naguib T, Yang SJ, Nasr E, Jorba J, Ahmed N,et al. Circulation of endemic type 2 vaccine-derived poliovirus in Egypt from 1983 to 1993.J Virol. 2003 Aug;77(15):8366-77.

21. Kew O, Morris-Glasgow V, Landaverde M, Burns C, Shaw J, Garib Z, et al. Outbreak of poliomyelitis in Hispaniola associated with circulating type 1 vaccine-derived poliovirus. Science. 2002 Apr 12;296 (5566):356-9. Epub 2002 Mar 14.

22. Chumakov KM, Powers LB, Noonan KE, Roninson IB and Levenbook IS. (1991) Correlation between amount of virus with altered nucleotide sequence and the monkey test for acceptability of oral poliovirus vaccine. Proc. Natl. Acad. Sci. USA, 1991;88(6): 199-203.

23. Chumakov KM., Norwood LB, Parker ML, Dragunsky EM, Ran,Y and Levenbook IS. (1992) RNA Sequence Variants in Live Poliovirus Vaccine and Their Relation to Neurovirulence J. Virol,1992; 66, 966 – 970.

Chapter 4 Jonas Salk and the Inactivated Poliovirus Vaccine

1. Smith JS. Patenting the Sun. Polio and the Salk Vaccine.W. Morrow, New York, 1990: p 61-73.

2. John TJ and Steinhoff MC. Appropriate strategy for childhood immunization in India. 1. Prioritisation of vaccines.Indian J Pediatrics 1980; 47:463-466

3. Fitzpatrick M. The Cutter Incident: How America's First Polio Vaccine Led to a Growing Vaccine Crisis. J R Soc Med. 2006;99(3):156.

4. Shorter, Edward. The Health Century. Doubleday, New York, 1987. Page 68

5. Kluger J. Spendid Solution. Jonas Salk and the Conquest of Polio. Penguin Books London, 2004. Page 35

6. Jacobs CD. Jonas Salk. Oxford University Press, Oxford, 2015. Page 24.

7. Oshinsky, DM. Polio. An American Story. Oxford University Press, New York, 2005: page 124.

8. Kluger J. Spendid Solution: Jonas Salk and the conquest of polio. 2006; Berkley Publishing Group, New York. Page 108

9. Greene R. The Concise 48 Laws of Power. 2002 Profile Books Ltd. Great Britain ;page 151

10. History.com Editors. Manhattan project. https://www.history.com/topics/world-war-ii/the-manhattan-project Updated 16 May 2019, Accessed on 25th Dec 2020.

Chapter 5 Albert Sabin and Oral Poliovirus Vaccine

1. Albert Bruce Sabin Facts.https://biography.yourdictionary.com/albert-bruce-sabin. Accessed on 29th Dec 2019.

2. Sabin AB, Olitsky PK. Cultivation of poliomyelitis virus in vitro in human embryonic nervous tissue. Proc Soc Exp Biol Med 1936; 31: 357-359.

3. Enders JF, Weller TH, Robbins FC. Cultivation of the Lansing strain of poliomyelitis virus in cultures of various human embryonic tissues Science 1949; 109: 85-87.

4. Youngner JS. Monolayer tissue cultures. II. poliomyelitis virus assay in roller type cultures of trypsin-dispersed monkey kidney. Proc Soc Exp Biol Med 1954; 85: 527.

5. Kopsowski H, Jervis GA, Norton TW. Immune response in human volunteers upon oral administration of a rodent-adapted strain of poliomyelitis virus. Am J Hyg 1952; 55: 108-126.

6. Melnick JL. Live attenuated poliovirus vaccines. In Plotkin SA, Mortimer EA (Eds). Vaccines, second edition. WB Saunders, Philadelphia,1994, Chapter 7; 154-204

7. Melnick JL. Problems associated with the use of live poliovirus vaccine. Am J Public Health 1960; 50: 1013-1031.

8. Melnick JL. Live attenuated poliovirus vaccines. In Plotkin SA, Mortimer EA (Eds). Vaccines, first edition. WB Saunders, Philadelphia,1988, Chapter 7;page 127-129

9. John TJ. Understanding the Scientific Basis of Preventing Polio by Immunization. Pioneering Contributions from India.Proc.Indian natn Sci Acad. 2003 ;B69 (4) :393- 422.

10. The relation between acute and persisting spinal paralysis and poliomyelitis vaccine(oral):results of a WHO enquiry. Bulletin of the World Health Organization;1976(53):319-331.

11. The relation between acute persisting spinal paralysis and poliomyelitis vaccine-results of a ten-year enquiry. Bulletin of the World Health Organization;1982(60):231-24

12. Esteves K. Safety of oral poliomyelitis vaccine: results of a WHO enquiry, Bull World Health Organ. 1988; 66(6): 739–746.

Chapter 6 Do wild polioviruses infect through the nose or the mouth?

1. Festinger L. Cognitive dissonance. Sci Am. 1962;207:93-102. doi:10.1038/scientificamerican1062-93.

2. Kuhn TS. The structure of scientific revolutions. University of Chicago Press, Chicago 1996.

3.   John TJ. Common strategy and flexible tactics in our war on polioviruses. Public Health Rev. 1993;94(21):151–2.

4.   John TJ. Can we eradicate poliomyelitis? In: Sachdev HPS, Choudhury P, editors. Frontiers in pediatrics. New Delhi: Jaypee Bros; 1996. pp. 76–90.

5.   John TJ. Anomalous observations on IPV and OPV vaccination. *Dev Biol (Basel)*. 2001;105:197-208.

6.   Proceedings of the Symposium: Strategies for world-wide control of poliomyelitis and eradication of the poliovirus from the human population, with application for elimination of polio in Europe. Public Health Reviews, volume 21, numbers 1-2, 1993/94, ISSN 0301-04 22.

7.   Brown F. "Progress in polio eradication: vaccine strategies for the end game. Paris, France, 28-30 June 2000 Proceedings."*Dev Biol (Basel)*,no.105, 2001.

8.   Wood DJ. Possible strategies for stopping immunization. Brown F (Ed) Progress in polio eradication: vaccine strategies for the end game. Paris, France, 28-30 June 2000. Proceedings.Dev Biol (Basel); 105: 159.

9.   Plotkin SA, Vidor E. Poliovirus vaccine – inactivated. In Plotkin SA, Orenstein WA, Offit PA. Vaccines, Fourth Edition, Saunders, Philadelphia, 2004; pp 625-649.

10.   Melnick JL. Live attenuated poliovirus vaccines. In Plotkin SA, Mortimer EA (Eds). Vaccines, second edition. WB Saunders, Philadelphia,1994, Chapter 7; 154-204.

11.   Oshinsky, DM. Polio. An American Story. Oxford University Press, New York, 2005: pages 8,9,11,16,22,24,85,86

12.   [No authors].The relation between acute persisting spinal paralysis and poliomyelitis vaccine (oral): results of a WHO enquiry. Bull World Health Organ. 1976;53(4):319-31

13.   Smith JS. Patenting the Sun. Polio and the Salk Vaccine. Bantam Doubleday Dell Publishing Group, New York, 1990: pages 13,85,86.

14. Martinez-Bakker M, King AA, Rohani P. Unravelling the transmission ecology of polio. PLoS Biol 2015; 13(6): e1002172. doi 10. 1371/journal. Pbio. 1002172

15. Arita I. A scenario for polio eradication. In Progress in Polio Eradication: Vaccine Strategies for the End Game. Dev Biol. Basel, Karger. 2001; 105: 33-40.

16. WHO.Polio vaccines: WHO position paper, January 2014--recommendations.Vaccine. 2014 Jul 16;32(33):4117-8. doi: 10.1016/j.vaccine.2014.04.023. Epub 2014 Apr 24.

17. WHO.Polio vaccines: WHO position paper, March 2016-recommendations.Vaccine. 2017 Mar 1;35(9):1197-1199. doi: 10.1016/j.vaccine.2016.11.017. Epub 2016 Nov 25.

18. Feldman RA, Christopher S, George S, Kamath KR, John TJ. Infection and disease in a group of South Indian families. 3. Virological methods and a report of the frequency of enteroviral infection in preschool children. *Am J Epidemiol.* 1970;92(6):357-366. doi:10.1093/oxfordjournals.aje.a121218.

19. Atkinson W, Wolfde C (Editors) in Epidemiology and prevention of vaccine-preventable diseases. Department of Health and Human Services Centers for Disease Control and Prevention, seventh edition, 2002: page 72.

20. Patriarca PA. Poliomyelitis in selected Asian and African countries. Public Health Rev.1993/94;21: 91-98.

21. Kim-Farley RJ, Rutherford G, Lichfield P et al. Outbreak of paralytic poliomyelitis in Taiwan. Lancet 1984; 2: 1322-1324.

22. John TJ. Poliomyelitis in Taiwan. Lessons for developing countries (Letter). Lancet 1985; 1: 872.

23. Otten MW, Deming MS, Jaiteh KA et al. Epidemic poliomyelitis in The Gambia following the control of poliomyelitis as an endemic disease. Am J Epidemiol 1992; 135: 381-392.

24. Sutter RW, Patriarca PA, Brogan S et al. Outbreak of paralytic poliomyelitis in Oman. Evidence for widespread transmission among fully vaccinated children. Lancet 1991; 338: 715-72.

25. John TJ. Role of injectable and oral polio vaccines in polio eradication. Expert Rev Vacc 2009; 8: 5-8.

26. Yaari, R., Kaliner, E., Grotto, I. et al. Modeling the spread of polio in an IPV-vaccinated population: lessons learned from the 2013 silent outbreak in southern Israel. BMC Med 14, 95 (2016). https://doi.org/10.1186/s12916-016-0637-z.

27. Diop OM, Burns CC, Wassilak SG et al. Update on vaccine-derived polioviruses – worldwide – July 2012 – December 2013. MMWR 2014; 63(11): 242-248.

Chapter 7 Proof of Principle and Country Models

1. Malvy DJ, Drucker J. Elimination of poliomyelitis in France: epidemiology and vaccine status. *Public Health Rev.* 1993;21(1-2):41-49.00

2. von Magnus H, Petersen I. Vaccination with inactivated poliovirus vaccine and oral poliovirus vaccine in Denmark. *Rev Infect Dis.* 1984;6 Suppl 2:S471-S474. doi:10.1093/clinids/6.supplement_2.s471.

3. John J. Role of injectable and oral polio vaccines in polio eradication. *Expert Rev Vaccines.* 2009;8(1):5-8. doi:10.1586/14760584.8.1.5

4. Platt LR, Estívariz CF, Sutter RW. Vaccine-associated paralytic poliomyelitis: a review of the epidemiology and estimation of the global burden. *J Infect Dis.* 2014;210 Suppl 1:S380-S389. doi:10.1093/infdis/jiu184

5. John TJ, Devarajan LV, Balasubramanyan A. Immunization in India with trivalent and monovalent oral poliovirus vaccines of enhanced potency. *Bull World Health Organ.* 1976;54(1):115-117.

6. el-Sayed N, el-Gamal Y, Abbassy AA, et al. Monovalent type 1 oral poliovirus vaccine in newborns. *N Engl J Med.* 2008;359(16):1655-1665. doi:10.1056/NEJMoa0800390

7. Grassly NC, Wenger J, Durrani S, Bahl S, Deshpande JM, Sutter RW,et al. Protective efficacy of a monovalent oral type 1 poliovirus vaccine: a case-control study. Lancet. 2007

Apr   21;369(9570):1356-1362.   doi: 10.1016/S0140-6736(07)60531-5.

8. John TJ, Pandian R, Gadomski A, Steinhoff M, John M, Ray M.Control of poliomyelitis by pulse immunisation in Vellore, India.Br Med J (Clin Res Ed). 1983 Jan 1;286(6358):31-2.

9. John TJ, Vashishtha VM. Eradicating vaccine viruses: why, when how? Indian J Med Res 2009; 130:491-494.

Chapter 8 Ethics and Polio Eradication

1. Beauchamp TL, Childress JF, editors. Principles of Biomedical Ethics. 5th ed. New York: Oxford University Press; 2001.

2. John TJ, Dharmapalan D. The moral dilemma of the polio eradication programme. Indian J Med Ethics. 2019;4 (NS)(4):294-297. doi:10.20529/IJME.2019.060

3. AMM Payne. Studies on vaccination against Poliomyelitis with live virus vaccines. Bull World Health Organ. 1957 :589A:1029-32

4. Oral poliomyelitis vaccines. Report of Special Advisory Committee on Oral Poliomyelitis Vaccines to the Surgeon General of the Public Health Service. JAMA 1964;190:161-4.

5. The relation between acute persisting spinal paralysis and poliomyelitis vaccine (oral): results of a WHO enquiry. Bull World Health Organ. 1976;53(4):319-31.

6. WHO Consultative Group. The relation between acute persisting spinal paralysis and poliomyelitis vaccine--results of a ten-year enquiry. Bull World Health Organ. 1982;60(2):231-42.

7. Van Wezel AL, van Steenis G, van der Marel P, Osterhaus ADME. Inactivated poliovirus vaccine: Current production method and new developments. Rev Infect Dis 1984: 6(Suppl);S335-S340

8. Simoes EAF, Padmini B, Steinhoff MC, Jadhav M, John TJ. Antibody response of infants to two doses of inactivated

polio vaccine of enhanced potency. Am J Dis Child 1985; 139: 977-980

9. Lauren R. Platt, Concepción F. Estívariz, Roland W. Sutter; Vaccine-Associated Paralytic Poliomyelitis: A Review of the Epidemiology and Estimation of the Global Burden, The Journal of Infectious Diseases, Volume 210, Issue suppl_1, 1 November 2014, Pages S380–S389

10. Oral poliomyelitis vaccines. Report of Special Advisory Committee on Oral Poliomyelitis Vaccines to the Surgeon General of the Public Health Service. JAMA 1964;190:161-4.

11. Simoes EAF, John TJ. Antibody response of seronegative infants to inactivated poliovirus vaccine of enhanced potency. J Biol Standard 1986: 14; 127-131

12. John TJ. Understanding the scientific basis of preventing polio by immunization. Pioneering contributions from India. Proc Indian National Sci Acad B 69,2003;393-422.

13. Scrabanek P. Why is preventive medicine exempted from ethical constraints? J Med Ethics1990; 16(4): 187-190 doi: 10.1136/jme.16.4.187

14. Isaacs D.An ethical framework for public health immunisation programs.N S W Public Health Bull. 2012 May-Jun;23(5-6):111-5.

15. Kass NE. An ethics framework for public health. Am J Public Health. 2001;91(11):1776–1782. doi:10.2105/ajph.91.11.1776

16. The relation between acute persisting spinal paralysis and poliomyelitis vaccine (oral): results of a WHO enquiry. Bull World Health Organ. 1976;53(4):319-31. AMM Payne. Studies on vaccination against Poliomyelitis with live virus vaccines. Bull World Health Organ. 1957 :589A:1029-32

17. Lauren R. Platt, Concepción F. Estívariz, Roland W. Sutter; Vaccine-Associated Paralytic Poliomyelitis: A Review of the Epidemiology and Estimation of the Global Burden, The Journal of Infectious Diseases, Volume 210, Issue suppl_1, 1 November 2014, Pages S380–S389

18. WHO. Global Vaccine Safety. Information Sheet: Observed Rate of Vaccine Reactiopns. Polio Vaccines.

19. WHO.Report of the 1st meeting of the Global Commission for the Certification of the Eradication of Poliomyelitis. Geneva: World Health Organization; 1995. WHO document WHO/EPI/GEN/95.6.

20. SAGE Polio Working Group. Appraisal of options for certification of global poliovirus eradication. 23 Aug 2018.Available from:https://www.who.int/immunization/sage/meetings/2018/october/3_Appraisal_of_options_for_global_polio_certification.pdf

21. Price MR, Williams TC.When Doing Wrong Feels So Right: Normalization of Deviance.J Patient Saf. 2018 Mar;14(1):1-2. doi: 10.1097/PTS.0000000000000157.

22. WHO.Polio outbreak in Papua New Guinea. Available from https://www.who.int/westernpacific/emergencies/papua-new-guinea-poliovirus-outbreak. Accessed on 13th April 2018

23. AMM Payne. Studies on vaccination against Poliomyelitis with live virus vaccines. Bull World Health Organ. 1957 :589A:1029-32

24. Leone S.Sierra Leone investigates isolation of poliovirus type 2. reliefweb. posted 17 Dec 2020. Avaialble from https://reliefweb.int/report/sierra-leone/sierra-leone-investigates-isolation-poliovirus-type-2 accessed on 20 Dec. 2020

25. Mbaeyi C, Wadood ZM, Moran T; MJourn, Ather F, Stehling-Ariza T, et al.Strategic Response to an Outbreak of Circulating Vaccine-Derived Poliovirus Type 2 - Syria, 2017-2018.MMWR Morb Mortal Wkly Rep. 2018 Jun 22;67(24):690-694. doi: 10.15585/mmwr.mm6724a5

26. John TJ. Vaccine-associated paralytic polio in India. Bull World Health Organ. 2002; 80(11): 917. Epub 2002 Dec 3

27. Platt LR, Estívariz CF, Sutter RW. Vaccine-associated paralytic poliomyelitis: a review of the epidemiology and estimation of the global burden. J Infect Dis. 2014 Nov 1;210 Suppl 1:S380-9. doi: 10.1093/infdis/jiu184

28. Global Polio Eradication Initiative. Update on vaccine supply. Geneva: WHO; 2017 Apr [cited 2019 Oct 7]. Available from https://www.who.int/immunization/sage/meetings/2017/april/Changblanc_Polio_Vaccine_Supply_Update_SAGE_April2017.pdf?ua=1

29. United Nations. Population. Geneva: UNO; date unknown [cited 2019 Oct 7]. Available from https://www.un.org/en/sections/issues-depth/population/

30. Jorba J, Diop OM, Iber J, Henderson E, Zhao K, Sutter RW, Wassilak SGF, Burns CC. Update on vaccine-derived polioviruses - worldwide, January 2017-June 2018.MMWR Morb Mortal Wkly Rep. 2018 Oct 26;67(42):1189-94. doi: 10.15585/mmwr.mm6742(2018)

31. Jorba J, Diop OM, Iber J, Henderson E, Sutter RW, Wassilak SGF, Burns CC. Update on vaccine-derived polioviruses - worldwide, January 2016- June 2017. MMWR Morb Mortal Wkly Rep. 2017 Nov 3;66(43):1185-91. doi: 10.15585/mmwr.mm6643a6

32. Jorba J, Diop OM, Iber J, Sutter RW, Wassilak SG, Burns CC. Update on vaccine-derived polioviruses - worldwide, January 2015-May 2016. MMWR Morb Mortal Wkly Rep. 2016 Aug 5; 65(30):763-9. doi:10.15585/mmwr.mm6530a3

33. Diop OM, Burns CC, Sutter RW, Wassilak SG, Kew OM. Centers for Disease Control and Prevention (CDC). Update on vaccine-derived polioviruses- worldwide, January 2014 - March 2015. MMWR Morb Mortal Wkly Rep. 2015 Jun 19;64(23):640-6.

34. Global Polio Eradication Initiative. Polio as of 24th April 2019.Geneva:WHO; 2017 [cited 2019 Oct 7]. Available from

https://reliefweb.int/sites/reliefweb.int/files/resources/Thi
s%20Week%20%E2%80%93%20GPEI_72.pdf

35. Global Polio Eradication Initiative. Polio as of 26 September 2018. Geneva: WHO; 2018 [cited 2019 Oct 7]. Available from
https://reliefweb.int/sites/reliefweb.int/files/resources/Thi
s%20Week%20%E2%80%93%20GPEI_55.pdf

36. Global Polio Eradication Initiative. Polio this week as of 15 November 2017. Geneva: WHO; 2017 [cited 2019 Oct 7]. Available from
https://reliefweb.int/sites/reliefweb.int/files/resources/Thi
s%20Week%20%E2%80%93%20GPEI_26.pdf

37. Rotary International. End polio now. 2016 review. Bowenrotary.com. 2017 Jan 28[cited 2019 Oct 7]. Available from http://bowenrotary.com/2017/01/rotary-end-polio-now-year-2016-review/

38. Global Polio Eradication Initiative. Polio this week as of 30 September 2015. Geneva: WHO; 2015 [cited 2019 Oct 7]. Available from
https://reliefweb.int/sites/reliefweb.int/files/resources/Pol
io%20this%20week%2029092015_0.pdf

39. Bill and Melinda Gates Foundation. Polio strategy Overview. Available from:https://www.gatesfoundation.org/what-we-do/global-development/polio

40. Bart KJ, Foulds P, Patriarca P. Global eradication of poliomyelitis: Benefit-cost analysis. Bulletin of the World Health Organization 1996;74(1):35-45

41. Vulnerability (definition). Lexico.Available from https://www.lexico.com/definition/vulnerability Accessed on 13th Jan 2020.

42. Waisel DB.Vulnerable populations in healthcare.Curr Opin Anaesthesiol. 2013 Apr;26(2):186-92. doi: 10.1097/ACO.0b013e32835e8c17.

43. Reyes v.Wyeth Laboratories.United States Court of Appeals, Fifth Circuit,498 F.2d 1264 (5th Cir. 1974).Available from https://casetext.com/case/reyes-v-wyeth-laboratories

44. MacDonald NE; SAGE Working Group on Vaccine Hesitancy. Vaccine hesitancy: Definition, scope and determinants. Vaccine. 2015;33(34):4161-4164. doi:10.1016/j.vaccine.2015.04.036

45. John TJ and Dharmapalan D. Fighting Polio in Pakistan. In Hindu 02 May 2019. Available from https://www.thehindu.com/opinion/op-ed/fighting-polio-in-pakistan/article27004837.ece

Chapter 9 Wandering in the wilderness

1. Chumakov KM, Powers LB, Noonan KE, Roninson IB, Levenbook IS. Correlation between amount of virus with altered nucleotide sequence and the monkey test for acceptability of oral poliovirus vaccine. Proceedings of the National Academy of Science 1991; 88: 199-203.

2. Chumakov KM, Norwood LP, Parker ML, Dragunsky EM, Ron T, Levenbook IS. RN. A sequence variants in live poliovirus vaccine and their relation to neurovirulence. J Virol 1992; 66: 966-970.

3. John TJ. Two good reasons why type 2 virus should be dropped from OPV. Lancet 2004;364 (9446):1666.

Chapter 10 The Way Forward, Creating a Polio-free World

1. John TJ Immunisation against polioviruses in developing countries Rev Med Virol 1993; 3: 149-160.

2. John TJ Can we eradicate poliomyelitis? In: HPS Sachdev, P Choudhury (Eds). *Frontiers in Pediatrics*. 1996. Jaypee Brothers, New Delhi; pp76-90.

3. John TJ Polio vaccine strategies for the end game Lancet 2000; 356: 1682-1683.

4. John TJ. Oral polio vaccine: how safe is safe? Curr Sci 2000;79 (6):687-689.

5. John TJ. Anomalous observations on IPV and OPV vaccination. Dev Biol (Basel) 2001; 105: 197-208.

6. John TJ Vaccine-associated paralytic poliomyelitis in India Bull WHO 2002; 80: 917.

7. John TJ. Understanding the scientific basis of preventing polio by imunisation: pioneering contributions from India. Proc Indian National Sci Academy 2003; B69(4): 393-422.

8. John TJ. Polio eradication in India: What is the future? Indian Pediatr 2003; 40: 455-462.

9. John TJ. A developing country perspective on vaccine-associated paralytic poliomyelitis Bull WHO 2004; 82: 53-58.

10. John TJ Two good reasons to drop type 2 virus from oral polio vaccine Lancet 2004; 364: 1666.

11. John TJ. The golden jubilee of vaccination against poliomyelitis. Indian J Med Res 2004; 119: 1-17.

12. Ehrenfeld E, Glass RI, Agol VI, Chumakov K, Dowdle W, John TJ, Katz S, Miller M, Bremen J, Modlin J, Wright P. Polio immunization: Moving forward. Lancet 2008; 371: 1385-1387.

13. John TJ, Vashishtha VM. Eradication of vaccine polioviruses: why, when and how? Indian J Med Res 2009; 130: 491-494.

14. Garon J, Orenstein W, John TJ. The need and potential of inactivated poliovirus vaccine. Ind Pediatr 2016; 53(S1): S2-S6

15. John TJ. India's research contributions towards polio eradication, Ind Pediatr 2016; 53(S1); S38-S43

16. John TJ. Poliovirus neurovirulence and attenuation. A conceptual framework. Dev Biol Stand. 1993; 78: 117-119

17. Chumakov KM, Powers LB, Noonan KE, Roninson IB, Levenbook IS. Correlation between amount of virus with altered nucleotide sequence and the monkey test for

acceptability of oral poliovirus vaccine. Proceedings of the National Academy of Science 1991; 88: 199-203.

18. Chumakov KM, Norwood LP, Parker ML, Dragunsky EM, Ron T, Levenbook IS. RN. A sequence variants in live poliovirus vaccine and their relation to neurovirulence. J Virol 1992; 66: 966-970

19. Press Trust of India, Islamabad. Polio worker shot dead in Pakistan, over 100 killed since December 2012. Hindustan Times.[newspaper on the Internet]July 2017 July 27th. Available from:https://www.hindustantimes.com/world-news/polio-worker-shot-dead-in-pakistan-over-100-killed-since-december-2012/story-7nt0hXxatmuGNwrFe2wCsJ.html, Accessed on 4th Jan 2019

20. Khan OF. People set hospital afire in Peshawar.The Times of India.[newspaper on the Internet]2019 April 22:World. Available from http://timesofindia.indiatimes.com/articleshow/68997340.cms?utm_source=contentofinterest&utm_medium=text&utm_campaign=cppst. Accessed on 4th Jan 2019.

21. Feldman EV, Votiakov VI, Kardash LB, Gracheva LG, Teleskovets JF, Ralko LP. Summary of the study of the immunological structure of and spread of polioviruses in a population not immunised with OPV during a 3-year period. In MP Chumakov (Ed) Enterovirus Infection; Vol 14: Proceedings of the Institute of Poliomyelitis and Viral Encephalitis, Moscow, Russia. 1970; p187-201.

22. Korotkova EA, Park R, Cherkasova EA, Lipskaya GY, Chumakov KM, Feldman EV, Kew OM, Agol VI. Retrospective analysis of a local cessation of vaccination against poliomyelitis: A possible scenario for the future. J Virol 2003; 77: 12460-12465

23. Van Damme P, De Coster I, Bandyopadhyay AS, Revets H, Withanage K, De Smedt P,et al. The safety and immunogenicity of two novel live attenuated monovalent

(serotype 2) oral poliovirus vaccines in healthy adults: a double-blind, single-centre phase 1 study. Lancet 2019;394:148–58.

24. Konopka-Anstadt JL, Campagnoli R, Vincent A et al. Development of a new oral poliovirus vaccine for the eradication end game using codon deoptimisation. Npj Vaccines 2020; 5: 26 doi.org/10.1038/s41541-020-0176-7.

25. Smith J, Leke R, Adams A, Tangermann RH. Certification of polio eradication: process and lessons learned.Bull World Health Organ. 2004 Jan;82(1):24-30. Epub 2004 Feb 26.

26. Wahjugono G, Revolusiana, Widhiastuthi D, Sundoro J, Mardani T, Ratih W U, et al. Switch from oral to inactivated poliovirus vaccine in Yogyakarta Province, Indonesia: Summary of coverage, immunity and environmental surveillance. J Infect Dis 214; 210: S347-S352.

27. John TJ. Understanding the scientific basis of preventing polio by immunization. Pioneering contributions from India. Proc Indian National Sci Acad 2003; B 69; 393-422

28. Rabi Abdullahi v. Pfizer, Inc.Available from https://iilj.org/wp-content/uploads/2016/08/Abdullahi-v.-Pfizer.pdf. Accessed on 16 Feb 2020

29. Yahya M. Polio vaccines – no thank you. Barriers to polio eradication in northern Nigeria. African Affairs 2007;106 (423): 185-204.

30. Jegede AS. What led to the Nigerian boycott of the polio vaccination campaign? PLoS Med 4(3): e73.

31. Streatfeild D. History of the World since 9/11: Dominic Streatfeild. Atlantic Books; London. 2011, pages 308 onwards.

32. Hilary Butler. The missing key to the story. Reader Comments. Plosmedicine 31 March 2009; earlier published as Reader Response Feb 27, 2008

Epilogue

1. Vermaercke B, Cop E, Willems S, D'Hooge R, Op de Beeck HP. More complex brains are not always better: rats outperform humans in implicit category-based generalization by implementing a similarity-based strategy. Psychon Bull Rev. 2014 Aug;21(4):1080-6. doi: 10.3758/s13423-013-0579-9. PMID: 24408657.

2. Nagaraj AK, Nanjegowda RB, Purushothama SM. The mystery of reincarnation. Indian J Psychiatry. 2013;55(Suppl 2):S171-S176. doi:10.4103/0019-5545.105519.2

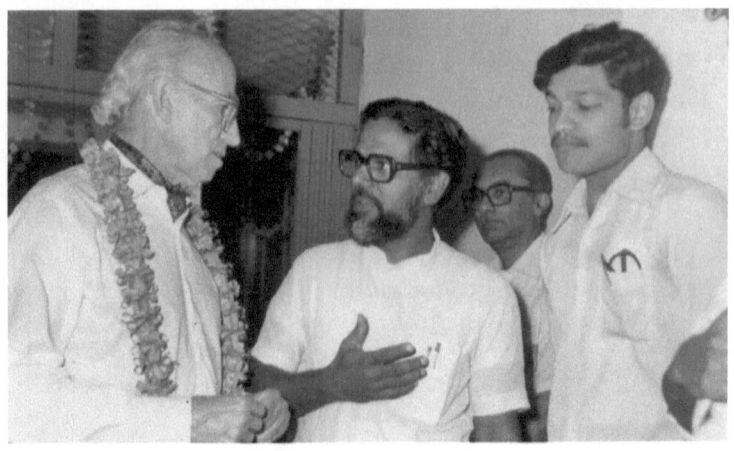

From Left: Jonas Salk, T Jacob John , Jacob Abraham and
Santosh Venkatesan.
Vellore, India; March, 1984 (Personal Collection)

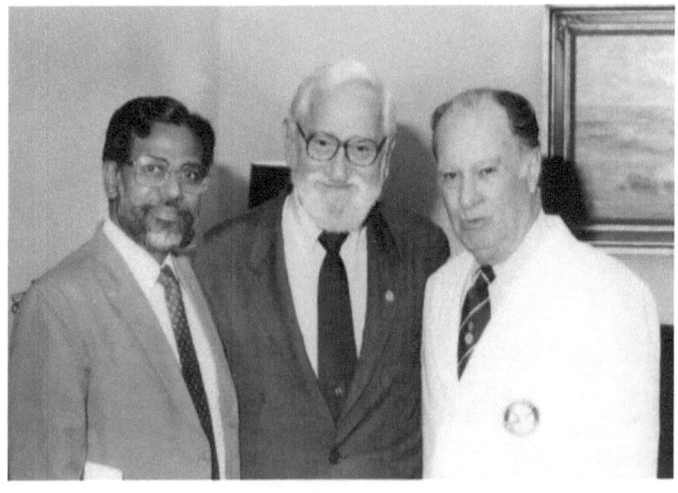

From left: T Jacob John, Albert Sabin and Carlos Canseco
Evanston, USA, 1984 (Personal Collection)

www.ingramcontent.com/pod-product-compliance
Lightning Source LLC
Chambersburg PA
CBHW020855180526
45163CB00007B/2519